WHAT PEOPLE ARE SAYING ABOUT PAUL NISON'S
THE RAW LIFE

"I have found Paul Nison to be one of the young new breed of people coming onto the health scene. He is like a young warrior determined to bring this to the masses."
—*Dr. Fred Bisci*, *Nutritionist and long time raw-food eater*

"Raw, Raw, Raw! That's the spirit! Go team! Paul, I applaud your effort and insight into helping others to improve themselves through the example you set and by providing this book as support. The testimonials provided herein will prove invaluable to anyone who wishes to make the transit to a healthy and more environmentally responsible lifestyle."
—*Dr. Douglas Graham D.C.*, *author, professional fitness trainer, nutritional educator and long time raw-food eater*

"Paul Nison is truly one of the most positive people I know. He is such an inspiration."
—*Angela Fischetti*, *fitness trainer and raw-food eater*

"The book Raw Life by Paul Nison is a great concept. It is awesome and his work is awesome. I have met many people who are into the raw food lifestyle. Paul is the first among them that understands the concepts and the complexities of growing into the lifestyle. His approach is fun and positive. His book is going to inspire many people to get into raw food and is not going to push them away. He should be applauded for it."
—*Gil Jacobs*, *Colon Therapist and long time raw-food eater*

THE RAW LIFE

BECOMING NATURAL IN AN UNNATURAL WORLD

Paul Nison

343 Publishing Company
New York, New York

Disclaimer to women

In this book I often use the term "man" or "men"in reference to "human" rather than to the male gender. In no way is my intent to disregard or degrade women. This book is for women, just as much as it is for men, and I hope all people enjoy it.

Disclaimer to all

This book is not intended as medical advice. When going on a natural diet, there is always some risk involved. Because of this, the author, publisher and/or distributors of this book are not responsible for any adverse detoxification effects or consequences resulting from the use of any suggestions or procedures described herein.

Layout & design: Enrique Candioti
Cover design: Paul Nison and Enrique Candioti
Artwork: Tom Cushwa
Editor: Arthur Goldberg

Library of Congress Catalog Card Number: 99-96140

ISBN # 0-9675286-0-7

First Edition, September 2000
Second Edition, April 2001

343 Publishing Company
PO Box 996
New York, NY 10002

RAW DEDICATION

This book is dedicated to everyone who has decided to follow common sense about health and life, and not listen to a doctor because society says so. You are not alone.

RAW ACKNOWLEDGMENTS

I would like to thank everyone whom I have met these past few years on the road to health. It is through our experiences, positive and negative, that I have gained the knowledge for this book. I am learning new lessons everyday. I look forward to new experiences and lessons.

I would like to give special thanks to the following people. You have all taught me special lessons about health and life that I will never forget. You are all champions! God Bless all of you.

Aldo Lafurio, Ana Vicenti, Angela Fischetti, Aris La Tham, Audrey Rochester, Brian Clement, Dave Klein, Dave Wolfe, Donna Perrone, Doug Graham, Enrique Candioti, Essie Honiball, Fred Bisci, Friends of Peace Pilgram, Gary Van Miert, Gil Jacobs, Glen Cohen, Gordon Kennedy, Habib Bailey, Jeremy Safron, John Kohler, Juanita Díaz, Justine Mastronardi, Lawrence Lyons, Madeleine Droego, Matt Grace, Morris Krok, Rhio & Lee, Roe Gallo, Rynn Berry, Stan Glaser, Steve Arlin, Tom Coviello, Tom Cushwa, Tim Trader, Eliot Jay Rosen and my mother and father Fred and Elaine Nison.

Note To Reader

Although I highly recommend a 100% raw-food diet in this book to help your body to heal and for you to return to nature, any improvement in your diet is excellent. Everyone's body is made to thrive on an all-raw diet. However, mentally only certain people can. This book will help you to achieve it mentally. Your body is willing and waiting to do it all the way. Keep improving your current diet and lifestyle. Enjoy it and have fun with it. That is the best way to succeed.

All the information in this book is based on the laws of nature. To understand what you are reading, I highly recommend when first reading this book to begin at the Table of Contents and read straight through.

In school you wouldn't go from first grade to college, skipping all the other grades in between. If you did, you would miss much valuable information. Consider this book the school of life. Read it in order, from front to back, so you can get the most out of it.

Also, throughout the book, when I use the expression, "cooked food is poison," I do not mean this phrase literally. Cooked food is only poison in the sense that it is not optimal for health, therefore advisable to avoid as one would avoid eating poison.

All the contents of this book are as up-to-date as at this moment. The laws of nature never become obsolete.

Contents

Contents

6   RAW SURVIVAL

7   RAW NATURE

8   RAW KNOWLEDGE:
Interviews With Long-time
Natural Eaters

9   RAW CURIOSITY

10   RAW TEST

11   RAW CONCLUSION

RAW DICTIONARY

RAW READING

RAW ORGANIZATIONS & RESOURCES

RAW FOREWORD
By Dave Wolfe

Several years ago I was discussing the topic of raw-food nutrition on a radio show in New York City. I remember it was a unique show—the host asking me questions every two or three minutes while he seemed to be reading or preparing other paperwork. In between the questions, I tried my best to provide the listeners with a barrage of as much raw information as I could get out. I announced my web-site address* and gave out my telephone number* as much as possible. I knew someone was going to call.

After the show, I checked my messages and one was from a young guy named Paul Nison. I called Paul and we had a great conversation. He ordered my first book and some other materials. On the phone that day he seemed a bit hesitant, a little bit shy, but very interested. I could tell he had been experimenting with raw foods, but had not gone all the way to 100%. Paul had a great friendliness about him.

During our conversation, I found out that Paul possessed a tremendous love for boxing! The "sweet science" has always been my own favorite sport, so I knew I would be talking with him again soon.

Neither myself or my business partner, the raw-food weight lifter, Stephen Arlin, author of *Raw Power!* heard from Paul for about 8 months. Then one day he called us and indicated that he had really made progress. He was overcoming a health challenge and was healing rapidly. He had worked his way up to 100% raw foods. From then on we have been in contact with each other regularly. Over the telephone, he also became a great friend of Stephen. In April of 1998, when

13

Stephen and I traveled to New York to do a lecture tour, we finally met Paul face-to-face.

Paul is a true New Yorker. His hospitality and kindness are amazing and he knows how to have a good time. Always the entertainer, Paul showed me some of the most outrageous clubs in Manhattan.

One of my most memorable experiences with Paul was eating durians (an exotic South Asian fruit you will learn more about as you read this book) all day and night for a few days and then playing a game called "What would you do for a million dollars?" We laughed about it for months.

Paul is an outstanding raw-food chef, with many years of experience. I was glad to see that he included some of his best recipes in this book. Prepare them yourself, taste them and enjoy them.

Paul is an avid learner. He is "Learning Man," highlighted in his book. He would not just jump into something without thinking it through first. In this book, he compiles some of the best ideas he has learned from the leaders in the raw-food field. He then integrates these concepts with his own experiences and philosophy.

Paul Nison covers every aspect of the raw-food lifestyle, from dodging the knockout starch punch to shifting out of the way of television. He shows you how to duck the butter punch and jab your way, step-by-step, to become a number one health contender.

When I sit in the first five rows watching the boxing heavyweight championship of the world, I know who will be sitting right next to me—Paul Nison, author of *The Raw Life*, the "Durian King," the great champion of raw foods!

This book has something for everyone. The interviews with long-term raw-foodists are especially insightful.

What excites me the most about Paul Nison is that he represents a new generation of raw-foodists; a generation dedicated to restoring the health and vitality of our bodies, minds, and spirits, and thus rejuvenating the Earth.

This is an inspirational and honest book. What a rare prize! Read on and become a champion of the world. Enjoy!

* **Dave Wolfe, J.D.,** *author of The Sunfood Diet Success System and Nature's First Law: The Raw-Food Diet. www.davidwolfe.com, www.rawfood.com 1-888-raw-food.*

RAW FOREWORD
By Morris Krok

Living the way nature intended is life's greatest quest and is the last frontier we must cross. This is the most noticeable omission in the philosophies, religions, sciences, arts, and cultures of the world. As a result, its absence has created the greatest controversy, confusion and complexities in the fields of health and healing. When we do not eat natural raw food when natural hunger dictates, we will suffer from every possible symptom that exists. We will even suffer from iatrogenic illnesses that are caused by using medicine or wrong eating to suppress every slight symptom and every sign of withdrawal, no matter how minor. Given time, this suffering will occur no matter what vaccines, drugs, supplements, or exotic foods we partake.

Man was never created to live in fear of the unseen, where goblins, ghosts, demons, bacteria, germs and viruses loom. A person living healthfully has no psychological problems, nor is his mind replete with beliefs, wishful thinking and brainwashing from irrational teachings and misconceptions from every conceivable source. We have been given a body in which every tissue and membrane and the entire vascular system is so sparkling clean that the purified brain is in a heightened state of awareness which puts us into a state of consciousness in which our true power lies. When you consider all the remarkable components of the human body—chemical, mechanical, electronic and structural—nothing is more profound, magical, and mysterious than thought: its origin, how it is stored, classified, categorized, and abbreviated, and how it can be collated and associated with other thoughts.

Though the body is intricately devised, it still operates on such simple principles that, providing we follow a few rules, we need not know the workings of all the inner glands and organs. The most important rule is that one must eat only when true hunger is present, and avoid eating by the clock just to appease appetite. When we follow this rule, we enable the intelligence within to do its work, with no interruption, interference or distraction. Since the body knows what is has to do in its own time, in its own unique way, a balance is created between assimilation and elimination. This balance is the true formula for health.

The body embraces cause and effect and makes many other concepts, such as food combining, irrelevant. This includes the beliefs that there is such a thing as a specific illness that requires specific remedies. It is because this conception has existed throughout the ages and has been given authoritative approval worldwide that has resulted in the creation of a mire that every deep-thinking person must wade through. On the one hand, we are told that fasting, or exercise, or vaccines and drugs, or supplements is the answer, and on the other hand, that healing occurs best through the combination of clean water, fresh air, rest and sunshine. When we follow this latter choice, we automatically invoke bodily processes such as peristalsis, osmosis, and the hydraulic pressure associated with the ileo-caecal valve.

As health, vitality, and the radiant rays of the sun cannot be stored in bottles, packages, or syringes, I have to accept that the latter view is the closest we can come to the truth. Over 4000 years ago, the yogis observed in their meditations and periods of intense concentration that to maintain youthfulness and effulgent thinking, daily internal purification in conjunction with eating raw foods * is necessary and is the highest and most noteworthy thing we can do for ourselves.

18

The system they devised, known as the six shatkarmas, is so comprehensive that it cleanses all the hollow organs, such as the stomach, bladder and lungs, as well as all the apertures, such as the anus, ears, nose, sinuses, throat and urethra duct. They based this method on the knowledge that the body has accumulated unwanted substances from infancy, which can be stored in the deeper tissues and which (as they are unwanted and not easily eliminated) perpetually feed our illnesses and our symptoms. This proves that the past's secret entrance and its wisdom is the door to the future. As man and his orthodox medicine do not understand the relationship between illnesses and the foods that one eats, he is constantly seeking after miracles. But the real magic is found when we utilize the seemingly insignificant intelligent and powerful logic that is found in every warp and weave of life, but is hidden to those who are not in harmony with or attuned to the realities of life.

---

* Those raw foods are foods which do not leave toxins, slime and other unwanted residues in its passage through the alimentary canal.

—**Morris Krok,** *author and long-time raw-food authority.*

RAW TEST
"Reality Check"

Before continuing, answer these commonly asked questions on health. Write your answers below or on a separate sheet of paper. After you read this book, answer the same questions again to see what you have learned about true health.

If you answered them the same way, you either got them all correct the first time (meaning that you did not need to read this book) or you answered them incorrectly again. In the latter case, you might want to re-read this book to see if you really understood what you read.

1. Who can keep your body as healthy as possible?

A. A Medical Doctor

B. A Holistic Doctor

C. A Specialist

D. Yourself

2. Cooked food is necessary to live a healthy life.

A. True

B. False

3. A vegetarian diet is deficient in protein.

   A. True

   B. False

4. The food you eat has no impact on your health.

   A. True

   B. False

5. For a happy and healthy life, a natural diet of raw fruits and vegetables is best.

   A. True

   B. False

"When you strive to seek the truth, truth will forever become your companion and you will never need to search for it again."

—Morris Krok

RAW NATURE BOY
About The Author Paul Nison

Until I was 19 years old, I ate the Standard American Diet (SAD). Then I received my wake-up call. I was diagnosed with ulcerative colitis. Most people would consider this a tragedy. I consider it one of the best things that ever happened to me.

Ulcerative colitis is not an easy illness to live with. The colon is achy and inflamed with ulcerations, sometimes with bleeding. It is accompanied by spasmodic and frequent bowel movements. The typical poor diet, increased bowel movements, decreased assimilation of food, and drug therapies all add up to malnutrition and decreased vitality, not to mention misery and a ruined life.

I experienced colitis flare-ups about six times per year. Every time I went to the doctor, she told me to stay away from dairy foods until I felt better. Then she increased the dosage of steroids she was giving me. When I felt better after a few weeks, she said it was okay to eat dairy foods again. I then ate foods that contained huge amounts of dairy. Sometimes this would be a whole pizza pie. Then the flare-ups came back.

I finally saw the pattern and cut out dairy products altogether. I was very pleased with the results. I became sick less often. After that I began to eliminate whatever the doctors told me was okay to eat. Eggs, meat, and sugar, to name just a few. I told my doctor I felt better without these foods. She told me that food had nothing to do with my condition. Since she was wrong about everything, I knew after hearing that from her, that I was on the right track.

At 23, I left my stressful job in the financial district in New

York as an office manager for a big Wall Street company, and moved to West Palm Beach, Florida. I was still having colitis flare-ups, but not as often or as severe. By seemingly sheer coincidence, I moved near a place called The Hippocrates Health Institute. I would visit the Institute often during my daily walks around the neighborhood. At the Institute, I learned about the raw-food lifestyle and about live foods. I immediately put myself on an 80% raw-food diet. What a difference it made! I told my doctor in New York about my improvement and she said that raw foods were not good for my condition. Once again, I knew I was on the right track!

Feeling much better, but not totally cured, I moved back to New York when I was 25 and resumed the stressful job I left. In New York, I met many people who had adopted a raw-food diet. I began reading more books on the raw-food diet and lifestyle. In a bookstore in Manhattan, I picked up a book by David Klein called, *The Fruits of Healing—A Story About A Natural Healing of Ulcerative Colitis*. It was exactly what I needed to read. I then heard David Wolfe of Nature's First Law speaking on a local radio show about the raw-food diet. Nature's First Law is an organization dedicated to spreading the word about the raw food movement. David Wolfe is one of the author's of a book he and his co-authors wrote called *The Raw Food Diet*. After speaking to Dave Klein and hearing David Wolfe on the radio, I decided to switch to a 100% raw-food diet. I also decided to join a raw-food support group. At that support group, I met raw fooders Matt Grace and Tom Coviello, and later, at a fantastic lecture she gave, I met Roe Gallo. The more I got involved with the raw-food lifestyle, the more positive my outlook on life became. Speaking to all of these people and seeing what great health they enjoyed influenced me to adopt a diet that consisted mostly of fruit. That was the final piece in my health puzzle.

Since going 100% raw, I have completely overcome ulcerative colitis. I feel better than ever and have become increasingly inspired about life. I quit my stressful job and began working as a raw-food chef in a vegetarian restaurant. I organize monthly raw-food potlucks, started a raw-food support group and I give lectures on the raw-food lifestyle to help others that have gotten their wake-up call.

I have recently traveled the world to experience the pleasures of new cultures and exotic fruits. Since adopting the raw-food diet, I have gone through several "healing crises." I am happy to have these episodes of elimination, as they are clearly my body's way of cleaning, healing and rejuvenating. I know the raw-food diet is the best way for me to go.

Just as I have, anyone can overcome any dis-ease or sickness. This book will help you accomplish your health goals. I can only tell you about it, the rest is up to you. I encourage you to learn from my experience and from other people's experiences. With a healthy mind, you can overcome anything.

*"You can lead a horse to water, but you
can't make him drink."*

*"Learn from other people's mistakes,
you will save so much time."*

"There is nothing stronger than the power of the mind."

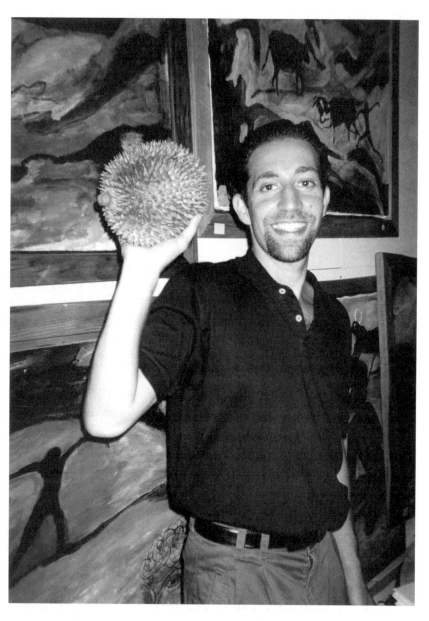

**The author Paul Nison with a "durian, an exotic fruit
from Southeast Asia.**

RAW INTRODUCTION

I wrote this book to give support to anyone who decides to improve the quality of his or her life. The information in this book is true and correct, based on factual evidence, unless otherwise noted. I do not claim to know all the answers or everything there is to know about health. Rather than blindly accepting common beliefs, I have made every effort to be faithful to the laws of nature. They are there for all of us to learn, and once you accept them, life becomes simple.

This book will help you to learn about health. I will explain to you how to strive to be as healthy and natural as you can be, fearless about health, life and nature. The book will help you to achieve these goals, while having fun in the process.

The raw way of eating goes back to man's first days on Earth. There is no mention of Weight Watchers or The Zone Diet in the Bible. What is stated in Genesis 1:29 is that the original diet of mankind consisted of "fruits and herbs" (i.e., green leafy vegetables.) Follow that advice today and you will become natural and healthy again.

The dictionary defines health as "The state of fitness of the body or the mind." As soon as we are fed unnatural processed foods, our health declines. It continues to decline from that point on.

We have all heard about calories, protein, and fat. If you ate the way nature intended, you would not care about any of them. If counting calories, burning fat, and eating high protein are so important, why are Americans who engage in these practices the most overweight, disease-ridden people in the world? Getting back to true, natural health is about preserving the energy of your body, which is accomplished by preserving its enzymes. Eating the best quality foods available and avoiding overeating will achieve that goal. "Eat organic raw foods in small but sufficient amounts and think positive thoughts all the time!"

Cooked food and too much food (overeating) will destroy you every time you put them in your body. Eating cooked and processed food is our biggest addiction. The longer you live with an addiction, the harder it is to break, and most of us have been eating cooked food since we were born. We ate cooked foods before we learned how to walk or talk. To regain our health, we need to avoid cooked foods and to replace them with the best quality foods available; i.e., raw and organic foods. In addition, no matter how good the food you eat might be, if you are eating too much of it, your body will become clogged. When this happens, your body will not even be able to use this good food. If you overeat, the food goes to waste; and in time, *you too* will go to waste. Never overeat!

Food, by itself, has no healing power. Your body does the healing. However, raw foods and a proper environment give your body the raw materials it needs to detoxify, to create energy, and to rebuild itself. Your body knows how to heal and is always trying to heal. The instructions for self-healing, in fact, are encoded in the genes of every cell in your body. As Dr. Hereward Carrington stated in his book *Fasting for Health and Long Life*: ***"Nature alone cures! All that anyone can do is to assist her efforts, and permit her to repair the damage."*** Trust the intelligence of your body and allow it to heal.

Most people have yet to touch the surface of good health. Clean and detoxify your body and you will become healthy. What doctors call a "cold" is simply your body working to get rid of waste. It is the effect of your body cleaning out all the unusable foods you have taken in, through overeating, consumption of poor quality foods and bad food combinations. Learn and understand what detoxification is, that way you will be prepared to experience its tremendous physical and mental benefits.

There is really only one disease of the body. It is called toxemia. Many doctors of Natural Hygiene have proven this in their work, but common knowledge of the way the body works, along with common sense, will also support this statement. In his book *Toxemia Explained,* Dr. John Tilden explains the definition of toxemia as "nature's effort to eliminate toxins from the blood." He goes on to state that all so-called diseases are crises of toxemia. His book elaborates in detail on the true cause of toxemia and how to prevent it. He gives excellent information about toxemia.

Anyone interested in learning more about toxemia should read this book. Simply put, the main causes of toxemia are overeating and eating low-quality foods. You are the one responsible for putting these foods into your body. Once you stop, and start cleaning out the remnants of what you have already ingested, you will begin experiencing true health.

There are several stages to toxemia. Medical doctors have named diseases for each of these stages. The first stage is usually referred to as diarrhea or constipation. The last stage of toxemia is what doctors call cancer. There are many stages in between. Toxemia is always reversible until it reaches the final stage, yet nobody knows when this last stage will occur. Even a doctor doesn't know. What this means is that no matter how sick you may appear to be, or how bad your disease may be, you should never give up hope or quit trying to get well. I believe that 99.9% of all so-called diseases are caused by your diet, your lifestyle, and the environment in which you choose to live. Toxemia is a self-inflicted disease of the body. You are in control of it. If you take care of your body, you will not get toxemia. Eat only small amounts of the best foods, think positive thoughts, live in the cleanest environment possible and you will avoid toxemia.

Dr. Tilden wrote the book *Toxemia Explained* in 1926. The information is still valid to this day because it is based on the truth. If today's medical doctors really want to prevent disease and cure sick people, they should learn about toxemia. As Dr. Tilden stated in his book:

"Medical science is founded on a false premise. Namely, that disease is caused by extraneous influences, and that drugs are something that cures or palliates discomfort. The term "medical" means 'pertaining to medicine or the practice of medicine.' Anything used in a remedial way carries the idea of curing, healing, correcting, or affording relief; and this doctoring is all done without any clear understanding of cause."

No one knows your body better than you do, yet most people would rather listen to the advice an unhealthy person just because they have a medical degree and wear a white coat. It makes no sense to listen to doctors; instead listen to your own body. If you do choose to listen to what others tell you about your body, doesn't it make much more sense to seek advice from a healthy person? If you went to a gym, would you take advice from and strive to be like a person who looked unhealthy? If not, then why take advice from an unhealthy doctor? Stand outside any hospital in America and you will see overweight doctors smoking cigarettes. What does that tell you?

Medical doctors know very little about good health. They do not study health in medical school, which teaches them mostly about drug therapy. If your car broke down, would you take it to a dentist to get it fixed? Then why go to a doctor when you get sick? It is absurd. Why do you think doctors call what they do a "practice?" The answer is because they practice on your body. Yes, practice makes perfect but many mistakes can also occur during their practice!

In today's world, people tend to accept what they hear on the nightly news, or what they read in the daily newspaper, without ever questioning it. People are brainwashed about health; they are taught lies and myths. Finding out the truth is the first step to becoming natural in an unnatural world. No matter how much knowledge you have and how hard you work, if your information is fallacious, you will not get the results you desire.

People tend to avoid the truth about health because once they realize and accept the truth, great effort must then be expended to change habits. Most people are too lazy to want to get involved. If you feel lazy, you already have a form of toxemia, as laziness is a symptom of disease. The truth will always be the truth, no matter how many people deny it or run from it. Here is a great saying from Mark Twain: *"Whenever you find that you are on the side of majority, it's time to pause and reflect."* Even back then, Mark Twain knew that just because you are different from others does not mean you are wrong.

Much of the information in this book comes from people I have met who have been living as nature intended for many years. And they have superior health and vitality to show for it. In this book, I am attempting to pass on their valuable information to you. Use this information to your advantage. Use the information that makes most sense to you. Then see what

31

happens. Many other people have also shared invaluable information with me, far too many people to single out individually. I've tried my best to pass on their knowledge with you as well. We can also learn from people with poor health. In fact, every person you meet, and every experience you live through, can be a valuable life-lesson.

Your goal may be to have a 100% natural diet, or simply to eat more fruits and vegetables. The key is to get started. Have you ever said to yourself that you know you should eat more fruits and vegetables, but you don't like the taste of them? In this book, I will teach you how to enjoy their wonderful taste so you'll actually look forward to eating them. If you eat 100% cooked foods, you will feel awful and eventually get sick. If you eat 100% raw foods, after your body cleans out the residue of all the unnatural food you have put in it, you will feel true health and an amazing amount of energy.

You must realize that the only path to true health is to take care of your body.

There are two ways to accomplish this. The first way is to just dive right in and do it. If you have the desire and feel that you can, then go for it! However, if you do decide to alter your eating patterns abruptly, beware! Making such a drastic change will cause great discomfort and will probably result in severe detoxification that will hit your body hard and fast. Take this advice as a warning. Although I do know people who have changed their diet abruptly and had great success, it can also be deadly.

The second way is to make the transition in stages. Your detox will be much less severe and easier on the body but it will last much longer. For most people, I highly recommend this method over the first more drastic way.

Attaining the Raw Life is a fight to the finish. Like two boxers duking it out, it is a battle with you and your new healthy life fighting against your old diseased body and its toxic life. When you win, you will feel like the world champion. Nothing will be able to stop you.

Whichever way you decide, never say to yourself that you can't do it. If you even think it, guess what will happen? If you fear anything as you proceed in life, it is because you may not have correct information about the object of your fear. Obtain this knowledge and your fears will disappear, because fear and knowledge cannot coexist simultaneously. Whatever you decide to do in life, be positive about your choices and you will succeed. Think positive thoughts at all times: You could. You can. You will. Put those positive thoughts into action and do it! I will help you. I will train you. Let's get started!

"To run with the masses and be stereotyped is to disconnect and dull that spark within that is always eager to ignite. Learn the simple truth and go free. Truth will free you from verbosity and irrelevance."

—Morris Krok

33

What the sport of boxing and the adopting of the raw food diet have in common.

When writing this book, I knew what I wanted to say, but I wanted to make sure I used the easiest and effective way possible to get my message to you, the reader. I chose to the metaphor of boxing because it is so easy to understand. Most other sports rely on other team members in order to succeed. In boxing, it is all you. The harder effort you put in, the bigger the reward. There is much more to the sport of course than just two people in a boxing ring hitting and beating each other, but for the sake of keeping things simple, consider boxing is just that. I am talking about fighting for what you believe in. There is no need to know all of the ins and the outs of boxing to understand this book. Just understand that whether you win or lose, the point is to be in the game and to make the effort. If you never step into the boxing ring, how can you even get a chance to win?

It works the same way with health. If you think "I can't," then how can you ever achieve your goals? Once you accept that you have to work hard and fight to achieve your dreams, you have taken the first step towards winning. Now close your eyes and make believe you are coming down the aisle into the boxing ring to face your opponent. With each step towards the ring you are stepping forward to achieve your goals.

1 | RAW TRUTH

The Opponents

Becoming natural is like the sport of boxing. In this sport you have to defeat other fighters to get a chance to fight for the championship title. This is your title match. And then, once you have won that title match, you become the new champion.

If you choose the first way of drastic dietary change, it is like diving right into the title match with no training. If you think you can win this way, go do it. Good luck. Be strong and stay focused. If you choose this path, then go straight to the title match, to fight Cooked Food Man. (Page 99.)

If you choose the second way, to make the transition in stages, you will go through difficult training and fight many opponents (habits to break), one by one. You must keep fighting and get closer and closer to the title match until you win it, no matter how long it takes. Here are the top eleven fighters that stand between you and your championship match for the title.

11. Illegal Drug Man

10. Cigarette Man

9. Alcohol Man

8. Legal Drug Man

7. Egg Man

6. Seafood Man

5. Meat Man

4. Poultry Man

3. Dairy Man

2. Sugar Man

1. Grain Man

Current Champion: Cooked Food Man

Only fight the opponents you have to. I have listed them in this order because this order goes from easiest to hardest for most people. Fight them in any order you like, as long as you beat them all. If you don't smoke or drink, you have already beaten opponents nine and ten. There is no reason to fight Illegal Drug Man if you have never taken or have no desire to start taking illegal drugs. It just puts you one step closer to your title match. If you are a vegan, you have already beaten many of your opponents. Add any bad habits that you want to break to the list. Then go and beat them. This is your own personal list. It will be different for everyone, but these eleven opponents are the most common.

To help you defeat these opponents you will have your corner coaching crew, which is your supportive team. In boxing, a boxer has his trainer and other members of his team at ringside to help him win the championship title. In your corner crew is Learning Man, Language Man, Willpower Man, Exercise Man, Resting Man, Change Man, Sunshine Man, and Detoxification Man. You will also have a sparring partner who is your friend. He is Mind Man and his trainer is Voice Man. You will also have a support crew to cheer you on throughout your fights. You will meet your corner crew in the next chapter and learn all about them.

You are on your way to becoming as natural as you can be and to becoming a champion. Beat all your opponents (break all your bad habits) and you will become the world champion!

After you become the champion, you will have to face new contenders. As in boxing, they will try to beat you and take your title away. You will meet many new contenders as the champion. A few of them that I mention in this book are Weight-Loss Man, Overeating Man, and Frozen Food Man. The longer you stay a champion, the better you will get and the easier it will be to maintain your title.

2 RAW HELP: Your Team And your Sparring Partner

In the sport of boxing, the fighter does not go into battle alone. He trains for his fights with a team to help him train. This is his corner crew. His corner crew consists of a head trainer, other trainers, coaches, a sparring partner and other members to help him. Everyone in his corner crew is on his team. They are his close friends and will do all they can to prepare him for his fights. You have met your opponents and now you will meet the members of you corner crew. They will give you the support and knowledge you need to attain your goal. They will help you break the unhealthy and unnatural habits that keep you down. (These habits can be conceptualized as your opponents and you must beat each of them to become a champion and become healthy). Each part of your team will help you tremendously, all in different ways. You'll now learn all about your team and how they will help you. You'll also learn why they are so important to achieving your success.

Learning Man A.K.A. Knowledge Man

Learning Man will give you the information you need to defeat your opponents. His first lesson is to make you realize that you have to unlearn many untruths before you can re-learn the truth. In the past, you have been led to believe that your opponents are your friends and they will help you. This is not true; they pretend to be your friends, but actually they are hurting you.

Learning Man has some friends who will help. Reading Man and Study Man. It will help you tremendously to visit Reading Man as often as possible. Read as much as you can. There is much to learn and there are many good books out there from which to learn it. Don't just read, study what you read, and think about what you are reading. The books you read will have new information that you will use to replace all of the untrue ideas and brainwashed material you have accepted for so long.

Once your opponents realize you have learned the truth about them, they know they can be defeated by you. The more knowledge you gain, the better chance you have to win your fights. You will no longer be the underdog. The information you learn will put your opponents on the ropes. (Confused and trapped. Not knowing what to do.) Your opponents are not used to being there as most people lack the knowledge (that you will soon gain) to put them on the ropes. With Learning Man's help, you will knock your opponents out of your life forever!

"You are never too young or too old to learn. The more you increase your understanding, the more doors of association and opportunity will open up."

—Morris Krok

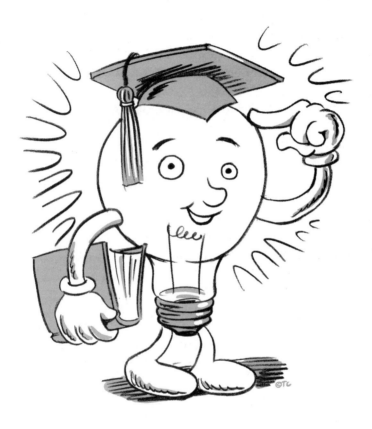

Learning Man
(AKA Knowledge Man)

Language Man

Language is much more than just words coming out of one's mouth. This is why you have Language Man in your corner and you must train with him.

The most important thing Language Man can help you do is to learn to speak positively. His motto is, *"If you want to achieve anything, don't doubt yourself."* If you doubt yourself, you are giving your opponents a chance to knock you out.

Your actions will follow the words that come out of your mouth. As an example, if you say: *"I will train hard, and then I think I will be able to beat all of my opponents"* you are leaving some room for doubt. What you should be saying is *"I will train so hard that I cannot lose. I know that I will beat all of my opponents."* That little change will make all the difference in the world.

Always speak positively. If you are really in doubt about something, don't do it at all! But once you proceed, use positive words and phrases like, "I can," "I will," "Yes," and "I'm sure." Avoid negative and doubtful words and phrases like, "I can't," "I think," "no," and "maybe." If your opponents start to beat you or you begin having doubts, say something positive. Even better, don't wait until you have doubts. Just keep saying positive things aloud all the time. It is one of your best offenses. Everyday, say at least twice a day, *"I can do this," "I am going to do this," "I want to do this,"* and *"I am going to have fun doing it."* Say it when you wake up, and say it before you go to sleep. That one sentence alone will make a big difference.

It is very hard to break any of your habits without Language Man in your corner. Train with him often. It will pay off. He is not only your corner man; he is also one of your best friends. He will be with you all the time. Remember that you can do it! You will do it! And, in addition, you will have fun doing it!

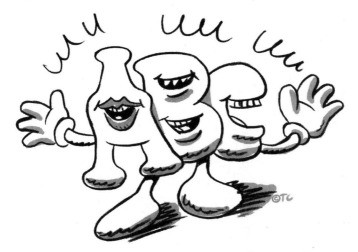

Language Man

Willpower Man

Willpower Man will help you to avoid doubting yourself. He will also help you get out of a negative frame of mind, if you ever do have any doubts. Every good fighter needs Willpower Man to help him in times of need. He is the difference between success and failure, between winning the championship and experiencing disease. You will never give up with Willpower Man in your corner. Willpower Man is the heart and soul of your team. No matter how bad things get or how bad you are being beaten, Willpower Man will not let you give in.

Other members in your corner will make winning easier, but Willpower Man is much more important because he will make sure that you don't give up. There is nothing in life that you can't accomplish with him by your side. Without anyone else in your corner, you still have a chance to reach your goals. It will be harder without them, but it will still be possible. Yet without Willpower Man, winning is not possible. You need him and he needs you. Willpower Man will push you everyday, every second. I cannot stress how important he is to you. With him there you will always be a winner. Willpower Man will help keep you on top.

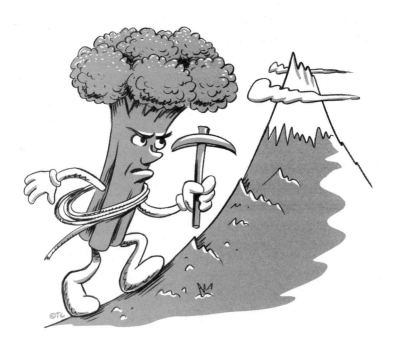

Willpower Man

Exercise Man

Exercise Man plays a very important role in helping you reach your final goal, to become a champion. As much as possible, make time for him .

"A strong, supple body can withstand shock, strain, and disease-building abuse to a degree that would wreck or kill the weak, flaccid, unexercised individual. Exercise is equal in importance to the cause of good health as good nutrition. Dependable high standards cannot be attained without it."
— Dr. William Esser, Natural Hygiene authority

The great thing about Exercise Man is that you don't have to use everything he teaches you, just some will be more than enough. Exercise Man knows many different exercises. He has many friends he will introduce you to. Some of his friends are Weight Training Man, Running Man, Calisthenics Man, Aerobic Man and Yoga Man. Be open to meeting all of them at least once, then you can make a better choice of which of them you like and will want to spend the most time with. Just make sure that when you do exercise, to exercise your entire body and not only a few parts.

Physical muscle-building and heart pounding exercises are both important. Exercise Man will teach you not to over-train or under-train your muscles. Once you spend time with him, you will learn what exercises are best for your body and the best amount of time to spend doing them.

Beware of Exercise Man's enemy. He is Burned Out Man. Overdo it and you will be sure to meet him. He will only slow down your progress. Avoid him at all cost. According to Exercise Man, you can do fine with a few hours per day of exercise, but be careful not to do too much. (If you are a serious athlete you could do fine with many more hours per day than the average person). You could even do fine with as little as thirty minutes a day if you wanted to. It is important that you visit with Exercise Man at least thirty minutes each day. Have a nice walk with him, or jog with him, or you could stretch or lift weights with him. Whatever you decide, remember to take it easy and not overdo it.

There is no need to focus on making time to spend with Exercise Man. It shouldn't be something you feel you *have* to do, but something you *want* to do and look forward to doing. If you have a very physical job, he will show up there anyway. In the past, people would meet him as part of their daily life. They would walk to work or go up stairs with him. However these days, many people plan time for him. If you make him a natural part of the daily activities of your life, (as they did in the old days) no specific appointments with Exercise Man will be necessary. That is the best way to exercise.

When I speak of exercise, I am not just talking about physical exercise. I am also talking about exercising everything you have learned. This you must consistently do. If you want, you can call this "practice." The bottom-line is that practice *does* make perfect. The best way to practice something is to exercise it. Whether this practice is mental or physical, exercise it to perfection in your daily life. No matter how much you learn in life, it would not mean anything if you didn't exercise it. *"Everyone has knowledge, only some people decide to use it."* Put what you learn to good use everyday of your life. Exercise it!

Exercise Man is not greedy. He will be happy just as long as he is in your life in some way. He will help you reach and maintain your goals. Stay in touch with him and some of his friends. If you do, you will be healthy and fit. You will be in good physical shape and ready for anything.

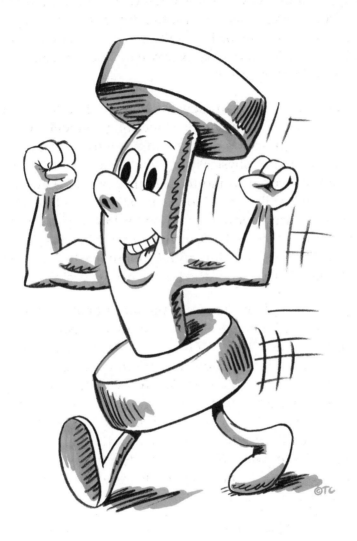

Exercise Man

Different type of exercises:

Stretching: Stretching will keep your muscles loose and fit. It will help you with all other exercises you decide to engage in. Stretching will prevent sore or stiff muscles and joints. Yoga is a form of stretching that is very good for the body. Learn the basic stretches for each body-part and practice them as often as possible. Twenty minutes each day is sufficient when it comes to stretching—more if you like. There are many good books available on stretching. It is important to have good form and to hold each stretch at least fifteen seconds.

Breathing: Most people do not breathe to their full capacity. Breathing exercises your lungs and your heart. Learn several breathing exercises and incorporate them in your daily life. There are many good books that will help you learn this. It is a good idea to practice breathing exercises during your stretching routine.

Resistance Exercises: Resistance exercises consist of any exercise you do that tones or strengthens your muscles. Weightlifting is a resistance exercise. Certain calisthenics such as push-ups and pull-ups are also resistance exercises. Resistance exercises are very beneficial if you want to put on weight by increasing muscle size. They help to build your body to its full capability. You can do many resistance exercises in your daily life naturally. Anytime you are lifting something heavy, you are doing a resistance exercise.

Aerobic Exercises: To exercise your heart and lose fat, do aerobic exercises. Running, rebounding (jumping on a trampoline), swimming, brisk walking, and bike riding are just a few examples of aerobic exercises. Increasing your heart rate in aerobic exercises strengthens your heart muscle. To get the maximum benefit, exercise for at least twenty minutes.

Resting Man

Your day starts and ends with Resting Man. You wake up in the morning with him, relax during the day with him, and go to sleep at night with him. He is one of your best friends. Listen to him, and he will take care of you. Resting Man is one person you should see everyday, without exception, for the rest of your life. You can visit him whenever you want—he is there waiting for you 24 hours a day. Always remember this little saying, *"For the rest of your life, make sure REST is in your life."*

If you neglect Resting Man, you will meet Stress Man and he could hurt you more than all of your opponents combined. If you get sufficient rest and good sleep, you will not have to worry about Stress Man. This is true but not as simplistic as it may seem. Stress can initiate a vicious cycle. robbing you of good sleep and good rest, which then affects your ability to manage stress. The cycle must be broken.

The body needs rest to heal itself. Continue to work hard, then give your body time to heal. The harder you work, the more rest you require. There are many ways to rest your mind and body. Spend time with Resting Man's friends: Relaxing Man, Meditation Man, Sleeping Man and Fasting Man.

Relaxing Man

Relaxing is doing anything you really enjoy, that is not strenuous to the body or to the mind. It may be laying down and doing nothing, watching an educational program on television, reading a book, playing a game, or going to the beach. There are many ways to relax. The main objective in becoming involved in relaxing activities is to "take it easy" and enjoy them.

Physical Rest

Don't confuse relaxing with physical rest. Once you understand what physical rest is and actually get some, you will become much healthier. Dr. William L. Esser, Natural Hygienist and author of the "Dictionary of Man's Foods," describes exactly what physical rest is and how to obtain it. I have read many books, and Dr. Esser states it best. Here is how he explains it.

"Physical rest can best be obtained by complete muscular relaxation which is most quickly induced by lying in a prone position. Many persons think they are resting when they are sitting in a chair and perhaps rocking themselves, or when they are merely changing an old activity for a new one. While a certain amount of relaxation may be obtained in this way, it cannot be compared with rest in bed. If a storage battery is to be recharged, all drain and duty must be removed from it.

To obtain the most benefit, the continuity of relaxation should not be interrupted except to look after immediate personal needs in the way of bathing, hygienic requirements, sunbathing, and brief walks. Energy is consumed by mental and physical activities of all kinds. Many more calories of energy are required to maintain the body in a sitting than in a prone position. Walking requires still more."

Mental Rest

According to many doctors of Natural Hygiene, Mental Rest is equal in importance to physical and physiological rest.

Dr. Esser states: *"The greatest amount of wear and tear on the physical organism is due to adverse mental processes and overworked emotion. To attain a high degree of mental rest requires considerable direction, concentration and application."*

50

On Dr. Esser's "Health Ranch" in southern Florida, one of the primary aims is to educate people who are sick away from their harmful emotional habits of worry, fear and emotional irritation.

Meditation Man

Meditation is so simple that it is hard for people to do. Have you ever heard that standing in one place is harder to do than moving around? It shouldn't be, but it is. In meditation, the same principle applies. Thinking about nothing is harder than thinking about something. Sounds funny, but it is true. That is what meditation is, thinking about nothing and giving your mind a rest. There are different ways to do this, but they all relax the mind and the body. By different ways, I mean there are different positions in which to place your body when you are thinking of nothing. They are called poses. You can lay or sit on the floor, or sit on a chair. You can even stand and meditate. Learning to meditate and relax the mind is a great way to give your mind the rest it needs.

Sleeping Man

Good sleeping is the best way to get physical rest. It gives your body a chance to heal and refresh itself. To help you get a good night's sleep, try practicing some relaxation techniques before going to bed. For example, if you have a lot on your mind, or if you trained particularly hard during the day, you will get a better night's sleep if you meditate before you go to bed. It is also important not to eat at least three hours before going to sleep. Your insides have to rest also.

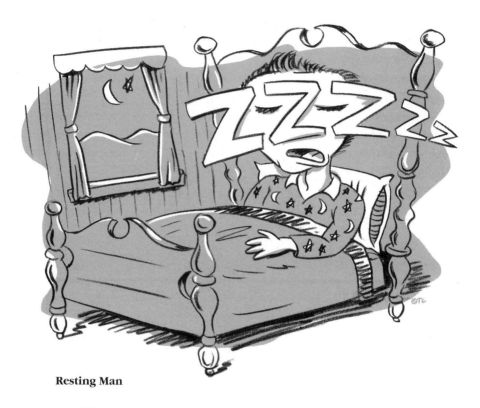

Resting Man

"Food doesn't give your body energy like so many believe, only sleep gives your body energy."

Waking up is an important part of good sleep. Learn to wake up when your body tells you, not when an alarm clock forces you. When you are awakened by an alarm clock or by any other unnatural means, you are shocking your body. That can be harmful. Even if you manage to get a good night's sleep, it will go to waste if you do not wake up naturally. When you do wake up, especially when it is naturally without an alarm clock, you should not be tired. If you are, it is a sign that you did not get enough good sleep.

If you are not tired, don't try to sleep just because a certain hour shows on the clock. If you are very tired and cannot fall asleep, find out why and fix the cause. (This usually happens because you are letting Stress Man beat you). Listen to your body. If you only sleep two hours and you cannot sleep anymore, don't force yourself to sleep. Too many people use unnatural drugs to put themselves to sleep. If you can't sleep, then don't sleep, because your body is telling you that it is not tired at that time or there is too much stress on your mind to get a good night's sleep. If your body needs 12 hours, then you should sleep 12 hours. Sleep as much as your body tells you to sleep. Average sleep requirements are between seven to ten hours a night. If you need more, make sure you get it. It is very easy to undersleep but impossible to oversleep.

The amount of sleep needed varies from person to person and will depend on many things. The basic rule is that the more active you are, the more sleep you will require. Other factors such as diet, environment, job, stress, etc., will determine how much sleep you will require. As no two people are in the same exact situation; everyone should honor their own sleep requirements.

In my opinion, you should sleep one hour for every hour you work. If you worked eight hours then you should get at least eight hours sleep. Twelve hours of work should require at least 12 hours of sleep. (If you work 13 hours and sleep 13 hours, that is 26 hours. There is not enough time for both, so you have to decide what is more important to you, a good night's sleep or working more along with spending time with Stress Man).

Stress Man

53

Resting Man says the more naturally you eat, the less sleep your body will require. This is because your body does not have to work as hard to digest natural foods as to digest unnatural foods.

> *"You can live months without food*
> *but only a few days without sleep."*

Fasting Man

The word fast is used very loosely. To fast means "to abstain from." When a person says they are on a juice fast, they don't literally mean what they are saying. A juice fast would mean they are not drinking juice. What they really mean to say is they are drinking only juice, as in a juice diet. An extended water diet (water fast) is the only true fast. It gives the body the proper rest it needs to cleanse and heal. All other so-called fasts will help the body to some degree, but only an extended water diet (water fast) will do the complete job of breaking down and rebuilding the body. The main reason for going on a fast is to gain these benefits. By an extended fast, I mean longer than the usual overnight fast we all experience every night when we are sleeping. An extended fast would be at least one day or as long as it takes before your true appetite comes back. There is a saying *"To lengthen thy life, lessen thy meals"* is so true.

Don't confuse fasting with starvation. They are as different as night and day. Fasting begins with the omission of the first meal and ends with the return of natural hunger; starvation begins with the return of natural hunger and ends in death. Where one ends the other begins. Fasting is beneficial, therapeutic, and heals the body. Starvation is destructive and harmful. Starving yourself has very little to do with food. A person can eat a lot of food and still starve if the food is of no value, as in the case of cooked food.

If you are interested in fasting, I suggest that you research its benefits and risks. There are many good books on the topic. Be careful and have fun with fasting if you decide to give it a try. (I don't recommend anyone fasting for more than a few days without supervision by a trained person who has personal knowledge of fasting.)

Physiological Rest

Fasting is actually physiological rest. I will refer to Dr. Esser's explanation of physiological rest. Once again, Dr. Esser's explanation of physiological rest is greater than anyone else I have read. It is no wonder why Dr. Esser is 90 years young and still in great shape. (For more contact information on Dr. Esser, his phone number and address is on page 176). Here is what Dr. Esser has to say about physiological rest.

"Physiological rest is best accomplished by the omission of all foods and drink except water. There is no function that is not intimately concerned with the digestion, absorption and assimilation of food, and with the elimination of waste products. This does not mean that the physiological activities of the body cease. It merely means that the metabolic rate is altered and that the various organs and tissues of the body are thus given the best opportunity to clear themselves of previously accumulated waste and debris than is possible during the most active stage of elimination. Elimination cannot be as complete and thorough when there is food in the body that must be taken care of. Clinical evidence supports the theory that much of the energy used in digestion is diverted to the organs of elimination during the fast."

These are just some of the ways to spend time with Resting Man. If you lose to any of the opponents, it is because they have beaten you; but if you do not listen to Resting Man, you are beating yourself. Make him your friend for life.

Change Man

You will have to make many changes to become healthy and natural. Change Man will help you make those changes.

*"The ability to change is the epitome and
definition of education."*
—Morris Krok

There are many ways to make changes in your life. Change Man says that the way that has worked for you in the past, or that you are sure will work in the future, is the best way to go. If you have not had success at making changes, or if you have trouble sticking to your changes, don't try to change your whole life in just one day. Little by little, make the changes you want. If you have many things to change and you try to alter them all at one time, you are setting yourself up for disaster. For example, if you have 12 changes that you know you want to make and you try to do all of them at one time, you will have great difficulty. However, if you make one change a month, in a year 12 things will have been changed successfully. Take your time and have fun with the changes. *"Change all negative things in your life into something positive."*

When it comes to changes, an excuse many people like to make is that they must set a date. Why should you set a date for something you can do right now? An example is someone saying, "I will stop eating meat on January 1st." If you feel you don't want to eat meat anymore, why not stop today? If you have the power to change something now but you wait, what is going to make you do it later? Time is one of the most important gifts of life, and wasting time is really wasting life—your own life. *"Don't put off until tomorrow what you can do today."* If you make a change, you can always fine-tune the change later. *The world never changes, only people do.*

Changes are good. They keep life fresh and lively. There are up-sides and down-sides to changes. If it is not a happy change, you must acknowledge this and learn from it, but do not mope about it. Enjoy all the changes in life. Most of all, enjoy life itself.

> *"Just because we are born into situations,*
> *doesn't mean we have to stay there."*
> **—Paul Nison**

> *"Many a person will not change to a better lifestyle, as*
> *nothing haunts him more than the fear of becoming*
> *healthy. Of course, he also thinks it is too hard."*
> **—Morris Krok**

Sunshine Man

Pay a visit as often as you can to Sunshine Man. He will comfort you and keep you healthy. Not only will he brighten your day, but he will also give you the solar energy your body needs to be truly healthy and strive to its fullest. His rays are powerful and healing. They help the body produce vitamin D, relax your nerves and lift your spirits. It is important to spend some time with him everyday, but remember not to overdo it. The safest times for you to spend with him and soak up his rays are from sunrise to 11:00 AM and from 3:00PM until sundown. As your body becomes more natural, Sunshine Man's rays will give you a beautiful natural tan and a healthy glow. Never block them with sun tan lotion and only use sunglasses to keep the sun out while driving. They are both very unnatural.

Mind Man & Voice Man
Your Sparring Partner & His Trainer

The person you will practice what you have learned with before fighting your opponents is known as your sparring partner. You will sharpen your skills against him. He is Mind Man and his trainer is Voice Man. Every time you train for a fight you will spar (practice fight) against Mind Man. *"If you can't beat Mind Man, you will never beat anyone else."*

You practice against Mind Man all the time. You know him the best. He might try to trick you every now and then, but if you can keep him in check and stay focused, he will never hit you with a good punch. He is stronger than any of your opponents. That is why you practice against him. Once you can beat him, the rest will be easy.

You can always beat Mind Man with your famous knockout punch. It is called positive thinking. If you ever feel you are losing or not doing as well as you should, just **"think positive"** and you will come back and win. Mind Man has many moves and tricks. His strongest punch is making you doubt yourself and making you think negative thoughts. Don't let this happen or he will take advantage of you. The way to avoid that is to always think positive.

Mind Man has a very good trainer in his corner. His trainer is Voice Man. He will try to get you to say negative things aloud. But you have Language Man in your corner as your trainer. He will teach you how important language is, what to say and what not to say.

Practice against Mind Man before each fight. He will show you what you need to know and what you need to watch out for. As much as you spar or practice against Mind Man, you should realize that he is your good friend. He wants to see you win the championship title.

Support Crew

Your support crew will make the path much easier for you. Having a good support crew is like having a match in your own hometown. Everyone will be cheering for you. Without them, it is like fighting in your opponent's hometown, where everyone will boo you.

Like water between rounds of a boxing match, find this support and drink it up. The more water you drink when fighting, the better; and the more positive support you receive, the better too. It will keep you going "full-steam ahead." Any bit of encouragement will do—you want as much as possible. If you look for it, it will come. You are not alone. At times it might seem like you are, but the more you become involved in successfully fighting your opponents, and the closer you get to the championship, the more people will start showing up with positive support. You will enjoy their company, but most of all, you will love their support. They will make life easier and more fun for you. They are the people who will be at ringside cheering you on at every fight you have. Appreciate and love them. They are part of your team today, and they will become your close friends tomorrow.

If you surround yourself with people who are constantly "negative," they will bring you down with them. Have you ever heard the saying "misery loves company?" Don't let them be your downfall. Being around negative people will only hurt you. *You become like the people you surround yourself with.*

Since the orientation of everyone you are around will rub off on you, you want everyone in your support crew to have a positive outlook on life—on everything in life they do. Search and find as much positive support as possible. All negative people in your life are part of your opponents' support crew. All the positive people in your life make up your support crew. People can visit Change Man and change if they want to; they can go from negative to positive. If they change, it is great for you; it means that one more person has been added to your support crew.

Your support crew will support you to the end. This is how you want all the people you meet for the rest of your life to respond; but there comes a time when you have to face reality. Many people are negative and do not want to change. They will not like what you are doing and they won't support you. It is best to avoid these type of people, but if you do interact with them, at least learn positive lessons from their negativity—observe how *not* to be like them!

If negative people do not want to use their positive powers, take their negative energy and turn it into your positive energy. ***Surrounding yourself with positive people is the key, when it comes to getting help from your support crew.***

You are on your way towards becoming as natural as you can be, towards becoming a true champion. Now, let us recap the most important points we have discussed so far:

1. You want to become as natural and as healthy as you can be. To do this you have to become a champion.

2. To become a champion you have to beat all of your opponents, the unnatural, unhealthy and destructive habits in your life.

3. You will have much support to help make your fights as easy as possible.

4. You must train against your mind before ever trying to beat any of your opponents (habits to break).

5. Once you do become a champion, you will have to stay on your toes. There will always be new contenders. They will try to beat you and take your title, but with your experience and courage, you will stay on top.

Now you are ready to go on to the next chapter and beat your opponents. Stay focused. You are on your way! Now get that title!

3 | RAW VICTORY

Let's beat your opponents

It is time to beat your opponents by breaking your bad habits. Stay focused. Don't give up. You can do it!

Illegal Drug Man

Most people know that it is bad to take illegal drugs. So when fighting Illegal Drug Man, you will have a huge Support Crew. Even the government will be part of your support crew for this match. Knowing all of this will help you. When times get hard, listen and you will hear everyone cheering you on.

Whatever reasons you had let Illegal Drug Man into your life, it is time to get him out. If you want to be healthy & fit and become a champion, you must defeat Illegal Drug Man. You cannot achieve your highest goals in life unless you are drug-free. You will have to work hard but your corner crew will help and make sure you win.

Learning Man tells you that when you eat foods that are good for your body, you will feel an euphoria that no drug can ever produce.

If you have been letting Illegal Drug Man seduce you because of depression, you should realize that taking any drug will not make your depression go away. It will only suppress the symptoms of the depression until the drug wears off. The way to get rid of depression is to find the cause of it and deal with it. Eating a more natural diet won't cure your depression, but eliminating unnatural foods from your diet in combination with eating raw foods will help you deal with the cause of your depression much better. To beat Illegal Drug Man, you'll need every advantage you can get.

If you are letting Illegal Drug Man seduce you into believing you can have extra energy through drugs, you should be aware that once your body is cleaned out and you live the raw life, you will have more energy than you ever imagined.

If you let Illegal Drug Man seduce you to get the feeling of being away from reality or you just like feeling good, a natural lifestyle and diet will help you accomplish that. Your lows if any, will be minimal. Being natural is like being high on life, and it is totally free.

If you are letting Illegal Drug Man seduce you because you want to be different, try living a 100% natural lifestyle instead. The way most people live these days, you will be very different. At the same time, you will be doing something beneficial for yourself. What more could anyone ask for?

Illegal Drug Man is a tough opponent to defeat once he has seduced you and you are addicted to him. You will still beat him however—just keep working at it and you will win. Language Man is telling you to say aloud right now *"I CAN beat Illegal Drug Man and I WILL beat Illegal Drug Man!"* NOW GO AND BEAT HIM!

It is now round one in your fight against Illegal Drug Man. Times will get tough, you will get cravings, so visit Willpower Man. Willpower Man will save you. Knowing that Willpower Man is always there will keep you confident. Know that you'll throw many punches and finally knock Illegal Drug Man out. He'll try to get up but he cannot. 1-2-3-4-5-6-7-8-9-10, you win! You win! You have defeated Illegal Drug Man. Congratulations!

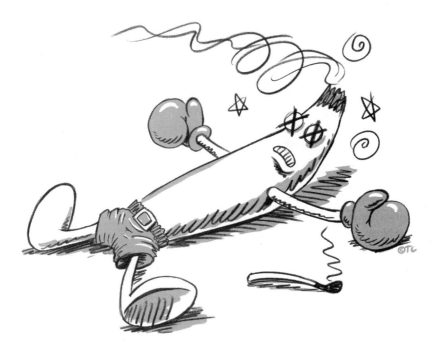

Illegal Drug Man knocked out!

Illegal Drug Man will always want a rematch. He will always try to hurt you, but you do not think about him anymore. You have other opponents to beat. Keep ignoring him and he will go away. The more you ignore him, the more he will stay away. He will try as hard as he can to get your attention, but when he sees that you are a new person and that you intend to ignore him permanently, he will stay away for good. Good work! Keep it up! Go now and beat your next opponent.

> If you take any drug that is unnatural,
> you will crave food that is unnatural.

Cigarette Man and Alcohol Man

For this match you will still have a big support crew, but the government will not be a big part of it, as it was in your last fight. In some states the government might not even be a part of you support crew at all. That is okay because, as long as many people are still cheering for you, you will be motivated.

It is time to beat Cigarette Man and/or Alcohol Man. During training, Mind Man tells you, *"just because the government says that something is legal, doesn't mean that it is good for you."* Many things the government says are good for you can actually kill you. As you face most of your opponents, you will see this more clearly.

You know how bad cigarettes and alcohol are for you, but you say that you can't stop using them, that you can't beat Cigarette Man or Alcohol Man. If you want to become a champion, you're going to have to beat them. Mind Man explains to you that nothing worth fighting for is easy. The larger the effort, the bigger the reward. Put in your head the thought that you can succeed and you WILL do it. Be positive about it. Leave no room for doubt. Now, go and beat them.

Learning Man says it plain and simple: Smoking cigarettes and drinking alcohol will stop you from being the champion that you can be. Stay focused on your goal. You are now ready for the fight... so go get them!

Round One: Smoking Man throws the first punch. He says that smoking will calm you down when you are tense and nervous. You tell him that once you become a champion you won't need to use cigarettes to calm down. You will get tense or nervous less often and when you do, you will have your support crew to help you. You won't need to smoke to calm down.

Now you throw a punch. You tell him that you want to be able to easily climb a flight of stairs like you did before you started smoking. That punch hit him, but didn't seem to faze him. You throw another punch and say that smoking makes your teeth yellow and smells awful. You hit him again, but you still did not hurt him. You realize that Smoking Man is easy to hit, but he is hard to knockout.

You continue to hit him with your knowledge about how bad smoking is, but still he will not go down. Nevertheless, you are confident you can beat him. You realize that if you keep hitting him, eventually he will go down. As hard as it seems, never stop trying to beat him. Never stop throwing punches and hitting him. Keep it up until you knock him out for good.

After all of those punches, you are getting tired of trying to knock him out. No matter how tired you get, don't stop. Keep hitting him until he goes down. He wants you to give up and keep smoking. The only way he can beat you is if you stop trying to beat him.

You continue to throw punches and they keep hitting him. You throw a knockout punch that your corner crew taught you to use just for this fight. That punch is the statement that there is a very good chance if you continue smoking, that you will have breathing difficulties or get emphysema. Even worse, smoking puts you at a higher risk to get lung or throat cancer. (Do you want to take a chance of spending even one day of your life talking out of a hole in your throat and not being able to use your mouth to speak or eat?)

You hit Smoking Man hard and knocked him out. You really kicked his butt. Always remember that statement as your knockout punch, and also that Willpower Man is in your corner. Then, you will not have to worry about Smoking Man beating you again.

Now beat up Alcohol Man. Learning Man tells you that Alcohol Man never actually beat you, you only keep beating yourself. The reason you crave alcoholic drinks is to satisfy your body's addiction to alcohol. Why do some people develop an alcohol addiction and some don't? It has little to do with alcoholic drinks and more to do with foods that create alcohol in your stomach. Cooked sugar ferments in your body, creating alcohol. Thus, the more cooked sugars you digest, the more alcohol you will crave. This is because when you are used to alcohol in your belly and then don't have it, you seek to bring some more alcohol in to get back to the state that seemed normal to you. Craving for liquor does not really exist. It is the alcohol in the liquor you are craving. This is why people addicted to alcohol, that have not had any liquor in years, never lose the taste for it. Eliminate cooked foods from your diet and you will beat Alcohol Man.

In his book *Nature the Healer* Dr. John Richter says: *"Cooked sugar will supplant the craving of your body for liquor because it makes a still out of your stomach, where a genuine intoxicant is produced. The liquor habit is a false craving, just as much of a disease, in fact, as rheumatism or asthma, and the way to cure this craving is simply to live on natural food. I challenge anyone to live on natural foods for one year and then take a glass of whiskey without vomiting. I have treated the worst kind of drunkard and cured his passion for drink by simply putting him on a diet of raw fruits and vegetables."*

Language Man tells you to say aloud, *"I don't drink alcohol."* Say it loud and say it proud. Say it to everyone, so they hear you. Say it to yourself, so you can hear yourself.

When it comes to beating Alcohol Man, avoid being around people who like to drink. They are all part of Alcohol Man's support crew. Stay away from his support crew and stay with yours. Your Support Crew are the people who will help you not to drink alcohol. They are all around you. You just have to decide to hang out with them. Remember this information during your battle with Alcohol Man. Now get ready to rumble.

Round One: The bell sounds. Here he comes. He is throwing all kinds of wild punches; beer, wine, hard liquor, and mixed drinks. Yet, he cannot seem to hit you. Now you throw a punch at him by saying aloud, *"I don't drink alcohol. I would rather have water."* You hit him hard with that punch. You follow up with a flurry. You say *"I don't want a hangover in the morning,"* and with other punches, you say, *"I don't want a beer belly," "I don't want to drink alcohol," "I don't like to drink alcohol."* Language Man has taught you well. If you just keep saying positive things, you will win. *"I don't want to waste my hard earned money on alcohol," "I don't want liver problems when I am older."*

You have Alcohol Man on the ropes. One more punch should do it. *"Did you know that most beer contains ground up animal bones?"* POW! You did it. You knocked him out. You are on your way.

"Raw food would be, if generally recognized for its merits, an invaluable ally of all organizations fighting the liquor and tobacco habits."

—Dr. John Richter in his book *Nature The Healer*

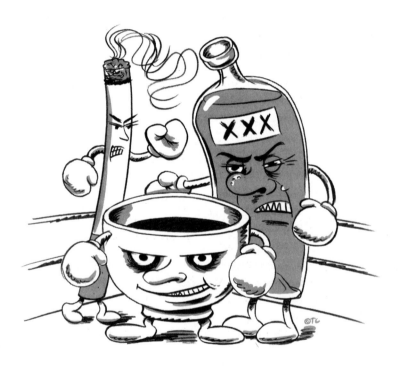

Cigarette Man, Alcohol Man and Coffee Man.
They are all legal drugs!

Legal Drug Man

The time has come to face Legal Drug Man. Although the substances referred to are legal, they are still drugs, and they are totally unnatural. Contrary to popular belief, they are bad for your health. To become a champion, you have to stop taking them.

Your support crew for this match is much smaller because most people don't realize the dangers of Legal Drugs. Seek the help of the people that do know and they will support you to the end.

To beat Legal Drug Man, you must know what legal drugs are. For the sake of this book I am using common convention in referring to legal drugs here*—caffeine, alcoholic, over-the-counter and prescription drugs.

Most people are addicted to legal drugs and don't even realize it. That is how Legal Drug Man is able to keep beating people. How can you fight against something you don't see hitting you? The first step is to open your eyes and admit that you are a drug addict. Yes, it does sound somewhat cruel to say this, but the fact is that most people are addicted to one legal drug or another, whether it is caffeine in the form of coffee or cola, over the counter drugs or even worse, prescription drugs. Any stimulant or sedative that is not natural to the body is a drug.

* In fact, all things unnatural to the body like meat, cooked foods, pesticide residues, etc. are really legal drugs in a more accurate sense of the word. As Roe Gallo says in her book *Perfect Body*: *"A poison is any substance that is not natural to your internal environment. Your internal fluids are poisoned when you ingest these substances. And what do you think this poison in your internal environment does to your cells? It destroys them! The consumption of poison perpetuates disease, eventually leading to death from disease."*

Here is your knockout punch. If you eat a raw-food diet when in a calm state of mind, balance your food in correct combinations,and avoid overeating, once you are cleaned out and have lived this way for a while, then you will have all the energy you need and will be in control of your life.There will be no need for caffeine or any other legal drug.Then you will beat Legal Drug Man and stop craving all addictive substances.

Now that you know all of this, you just hurt Legal Drug Man. He is on the ropes and has nothing left: one more punch should do it.You throw that punch. Here it is. If too many pills make people sick, why do people think one will make them better? POW! You did it! You knocked out Legal Drug Man. He is down and out for the count.

Now that you have beaten some very tough opponents,you should feel much more confident.Your Support Crew has had a major role in your success. With your future opponents, that will not be the case. People will expect you to be friends with your future opponents, and will start to wonder what is wrong with you and why you want to fight these opponents at all?

Most people will not make the effort to become a champion because they are ignorant or have been misled.They would rather live half of a life, but you know better.You want to become a champion and live a full life.

In dealing with your future opponents, remember what Learning Man and Mind Man have told you. *"You must first unlearn the lies and then you will have room for the truth."* No matter what people tell you, no matter how small your Support Crew may be, you know better.Training by Mind Man is an important step as he will help you deal with those people who look at you as odd. Now go on to meet your next opponent.

Egg Man

Egg Man is a sneaky opponent. He will appear in many different forms and hit you with many different punches. Sometimes he might even get help from his friends Ham Man and Bacon Man. He will do whatever he can think of to beat you. Be careful and stay alert at all times. You have been brainwashed into thinking that eggs are a great source of protein, low in saturated fat and that their fats are not as bad as other animal fats. These are all things that Egg Man wants you to believe about him.

Did you know that the yolk of an egg contains an extremely dense concentration of animal fat? In addition, eggs are the most cholesterol saturated food that people consume. One egg has ten times as much cholesterol as a hotdog. Egg Man has you fooled into thinking that if you only eat his egg whites, you will be okay. Albumin protein in egg whites is a concentrated animal protein, and eating it can cause calcium to leach from your bones, which may cause osteoporosis and other diseases.

Egg Man is also a very frequent cause of food poisoning in this country. One of his deadly knockout punches is his salmonella punch. This deadly bacteria is found inside egg yolks as well as in egg whites. The only way to make sure you don't get hit by one of Egg Man's deadly punches is to hit him hard, knock him out and move on to your next opponent. Egg Man can kill you. But if you hit him with one good punch of your own, he will crack under the pressure and break in two. Beat him and move on.

Round One: Here he comes, rolling into the ring. You have your Support Crew, and he has his. Egg Man's support crew is Cheese Man, Sausage Man, Bacon Man, Ham Man, Butter Man and Salt Man. They will all help him try to beat you. Egg Man doesn't waste much time. He throws a punch called scrambled eggs, and you decide to take the hit one last time. Just as you are about to get hit, Willpower Man tells you to duck, you do, and Egg Man misses with that punch. Look out, here comes a sunny side up punch. You never liked your eggs like that anyway, so you move out of the way. He misses again. You want to hit him and get this over with but you are having trouble finding him. Egg Man is very sneaky, he will hide and show up where you least expect him—in milkshakes, cakes, cookies, pancakes etc., in all different forms. Make sure you read all of the ingredients in everything you eat. If Egg Man is there, don't eat it. Now look out; he is throwing another punch. It is a hard-boiled egg punch. He misses again and this time you hit him. He is down and out. You did it. With one punch, you knocked out Egg Man.

Up until now, you didn't realize your own strength. Now you do. Egg Man is just the beginning of a long road to the championship. It gets harder and harder, but you can do it. Stay focused, remain positive and go beat your next opponent.

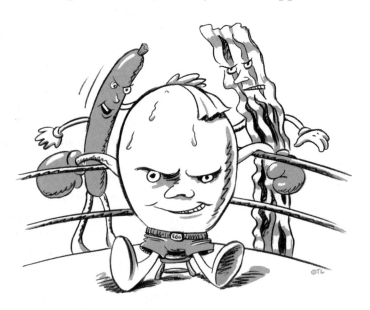

Egg Man with his friends Sausage Man and Bacon Man

74

Seafood Man

Of all of the species we consume, Seafood Man's family experiences the most horrible deaths by far. Imagine you were thrown into a tub of boiling water alive; or imagine that you were hungry, went to a restaurant, and ordered something to eat. You haven't eaten all day and you are really hungry. You see a special on the menu and order it. It takes forever to get to your table, but finally it gets there. You pick it up and take a big bite out of it. Right away you notice that something is wrong. There is a big sharp hook hidden in your food. You have bitten into it and it goes through the roof of your mouth, all the way up to your brain. It is the most pain you have ever felt. Then with the hook still inside of your mouth, you run outside looking for help and you fall into a swimming pool. Now you are drowning. You have no oxygen under water. You can't breathe and you are dying from loss of blood. I know this sounds bad. It is what a fish goes through every time one is killed. But before the fish dies, he makes a vow that he will hurt as many humans as possible for doing this to him.

Many people just decide to avoid eating any seafood at all because they know how the fish's life ends and they know about his vow. If you are one of the many people who think it is necessary to eat fish and still choose to do so, you have probably been lied to. You have been told that fish is brain food, that it is a very good source of protein, and that, of all the animals that humans eat, seafood is the least toxic. Learning Man explains to you that Seafood Man is one of the primary sources of pollutants and toxins such as mercury, dioxin, DDT and PCB's. Learning Man also tells you that seafood is not brain food like you have been told. Mercury poisons the brain and nerve cells, so seafood is actually brain killing food.

Seafood consists of concentrated protein and concentrated protein leaches calcium from your bones. You have been led to believe that Seafood Man's protein prevents you from acquiring many diseases. However, his extra protein is too much for you. It can lead to many sorts of problems for your body, including osteoporosis.

People think osteoporosis is a disease of calcium deficiency, but it is not. It is a disease caused by too much protein, especially concentrated protein, like the protein found in seafood.

To make matters worse, the people who sell seafood make it even more undesirable for eating. The flesh of a fish decomposes faster than any other type of animal flesh. To slow this process down, Seafood Man is sprayed with solutions of antibiotics. Some seafood is even dyed so the consumer will not see how bad seafood looks in its normal state. If you walked past a fish market and saw a purple fish with blood coming out of its mouth, smelling terrible with a big cancerous tumor on it, would you eat it? That is why the people who sell seafood turn Seafood Man into a pretty boy. They clean him up, cut off the tumors, wipe the blood from his mouth, dye his skin with coloring and spray him with perfume. Then they freeze him to slow the process of decomposing flesh. All prettied up, if someone now walks past the same store and sees the fish, he might consider eating it. And that's when Seafood Man remembers the vow he made right before he was killed. He will remind you of it and will be sure to hurt you in retaliation.

Round One: Here's Seafood Man coming right at you. Language Man yells to you "Say it now!" You say it loud so Seafood Man and everyone else hears you. *"As of this moment, I will never again put another piece of any kind of seafood into my body."* Seafood Man is down and out for the count. It's over! You win!

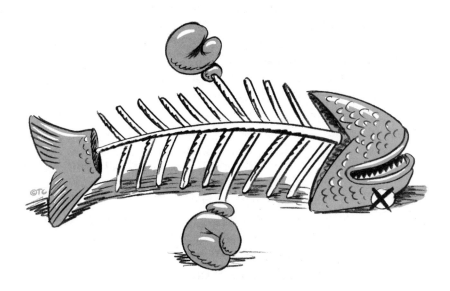

Seafood Man Down and Out for the count!

After the fight, Language Man tells you how powerful language can be. If you use the power of words in a positive way, it will help you tremendously on your way to the championship. If you use this power negatively, it will beat you up and keep you down. Always beware of the words you speak. To have thoughts is one thing, but to speak them is another. You just beat Seafood Man with a language punch. Congratulations. Move on to your next opponent.

Meat Man

Meat Man doesn't think you are ready to cut meat out of your life. He has a surprise waiting, because you are more ready than you have ever been. Meat Man is the one you have been waiting for, your toughest opponent so far. Your team will do what they must; they will have you ready to beat him.

Meat Man has many punches with which to hit you. This is why he is so hard to beat. Some of his more famous punches to watch out for are his hotdog punch, hamburger punch, steak punch, cold cuts punch and his pork punch. He is strong and he will try to hit you with as many punches as he can.

Learning Man tells you to learn about the pain and suffering that calves go through in the production of veal. Knowing this will help you to beat Meat Man. Male calves are castrated to become docile. In order to improve the quality of the meat, they spend most of their time eating—not only food, but other stuff that is mixed with their food. Sawdust and scraps of chicken manure are just a few things they are regularly fed. This is so they put on weight as fast as possible. They are also denied their mother's company and their mother's milk. The "tasteless gruel" fed to them intentionally creates a constant state of anemia. Many die from this physical & psychological stress.

Veal calves are also injected with many of the worst drugs known to man. The best tasting veal meat is supposedly pink and tender, with no muscle in it. For this reason, veal calves are not allowed to do any exercise so they will stay fat and not develop any muscle. Most of the time they are forced to stay in such small spaces, they can not turn around or even move one step. Older cattle have their horns brutally taken out of their heads so they don't hurt other cattle. They are given drugs to deaden the pain, but they still feel the torture. Sometimes their horns are pulled out of their skull without any anesthetic at all.

One of the things that make all animal meat so harmful to your health is that the animals are given anabolic steroids, testosterone and progesterone. When you eat meat, these hormones are passed on to you.

The trip to the slaughterhouse is not a very comfortable one for the cattle and other animals that are killed to be eaten. They are put into a trailer with so many other cattle that they can't even move. If they fall, which happens often, they are trampled to death. When they arrive at the slaughterhouse, they are taken off the truck by a machine. They are then met

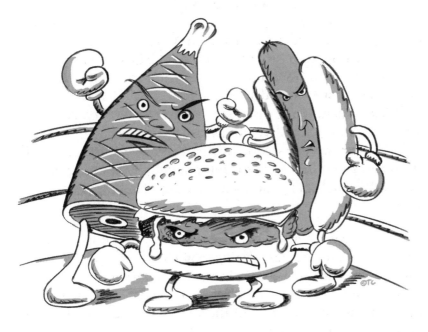

Hamburger Man, Hotdog Man and Ham Man

by slaughterhouse workers who sting them with a stun gun. Sometimes it is not done properly and the animals remain conscious during their deaths.

Next, they are hung by their necks and stabbed with a big

knife. Blood spurts out all over the place, pouring onto the floor. There is so much blood on the floor that the slaugther-house workers have to wear boots. The animals have their hides cut open and stripped from their body and then their liver, heart, tongue and other organs are removed. Next, the center of their backbone is split with huge power saws. The dead carcass is then hosed down with water and put in a meat cooler for a day. Their carcasses are removed from the freezer the next day and they are cut up, cleaned and packed. The re-sult is what you see in the supermarket, which is steak, ribs, hotdogs, hamburgers etc. Learning Man says the next time you go to the supermarket to buy meat, think about the way these unfortunate are forece to live and die. Think about the massive murder that continue, so you can eat meat. Here is your knockout punch. All the drugs given to the animals, plus the fear and dread that the cattle experience just before they are murdered, all go into your body when you eat meat. A part of this massive murder then contributes to your own death. When you go to buy meat, think about that. If you don't care about the cattle's death, you should, at least, care about your own. Learning Man tells you that humans are not supposed to eat animals. We are not designed to kill an animal and digest his flesh. Our bodies do not possess the physical structure that allows us to rip a chunk of meat from an animal's body with our bare hands and just chew on it. Nor are human teeth sharp enough to chew through the thick meat of an animal. If people only knew the process from which Meat Man origi-nated, they would stop eating meat.

It is not going to be easy, but you have Will Power Man by your side. You know that you will not lose. Now you have the knowledge you need to knockout Meat Man. Use this knowl-edge to knock him out and move on. You are in the process of becoming a champion. Keep it up!

If you do anything cruel to a house pet, you will be put in jail for animal cruelty. However, people who brutally kill animals everyday in the meat industry get away with it. They do not get jail time; they get money and grants from the government. What if these people came into your house and cut up your dog or your cat? Just because the animals that they are murdering are not house pets, doesn't make it right. What they are doing is still cruelty! It is still murder! There is a saying "kill one animal they call it cruelty, kill many animals they call it science."

"Don't let your stomach be a cemetery
for dead animals."

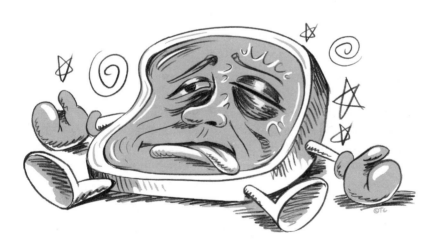

You did it! You knocked out Meat Man!

Poultry Man

You are half way there. Keep it up! It is now time for you to do battle against Poultry Man. You have been brainwashed into thinking that poultry products are good for you. This is not going to be an easy fight. Stay focused and you will do just fine.

The easy part about beating Poultry Man is that once you see how he really looks, you will not even want to be in the same room with him anymore. Poultry Man is not neat looking like you see him packaged in the grocery refrigerator. He is an ugly mean monster, with a lot of makeup covering his ugliness.

Every year, chicken, the most popular poultry on the market today, is made to look beautiful and scrumptious. It is after you purchase it that it becomes ugly. Let's call him Chicken Man. Learning Man will now explain to you what is so ugly about Chicken Man in his most natural state.

If you went outside to search for a chicken to kill and were successful, you now have a dead chicken. Take the feathers off and take a close look. Wipe away all the blood; disregard the cancerous tumors on the chicken or any other skin conditions that you notice. Don't pay any attention to them, or to the thick yellow pus leaking from the chicken's body. Cut around all of that pus and cut off any cancerous tumors too. Continue cutting until you cut off everything else that does not look good to you. (Don't throw away any of the things that you have cut off the chicken. Save them for later, so we can make delicious hot dogs with them. This is, in fact, what is used to make hot dogs). After you finish removing all the pieces that appear abnormal and diseased, wipe away all of the blood and throw the chicken into your freezer.

Wait about two weeks, then look again. The same chicken that you put into your freezer only two weeks before is a different color. When you put him into your freezer, his skin was a fresh yellow; now just two weeks later, it is a purple, bluish color. You wonder what happened? You are thinking that you never see chickens that have this color in the store. Learning Man tells you why the chicken changed colors. He says: "When a human dies and is frozen for weeks, does the body have the same complexion when it is thawed out that it had when it were alive? The answer is no, because their corpse decomposes. Well chickens decompose also." Now you wonder why the chickens you see in the store don't change colors. You realize if you want to do this disguise work yourself, you have some work to do. Just as the processors of chickens do, you can take some of the deadliest dyes and food colorings known to man and fix up the chicken to look as close to its natural color as possible. Now the chicken looks good, but what about that smell? Nobody would eat a chicken that smells like this. You go to work again and add more additives and strong perfumes to cover that terrible smell. You finish fixing up the chicken, just in time for your dinner guest. Now put that chicken into the oven then serve it to your family and friends.

Sounds disgusting? Gross, huh? I don't expect you to kill a chicken with your bare hands and to go through all of that trouble. The poultry companies who kill the chickens, turkeys, ducks and other birds don't expect you to go through that trouble either. They don't expect you to do all of that work, and they don't even want you to try, because they know that if you did, you will never eat any animal meat again. So they continue to make the process look as neat as possible. Up until now, they have been successful. Now you know the truth, so it is time to put an end to this mess.

Knowing all this about Poultry Man has him worried and scared. You know too much about him. He is starting to have second thoughts about fighting you. Because of what you learned about him and how disgusting he is, you don't want to fight him either, you don't want to even see him anymore, but you know you have to and you are ready to beat him.

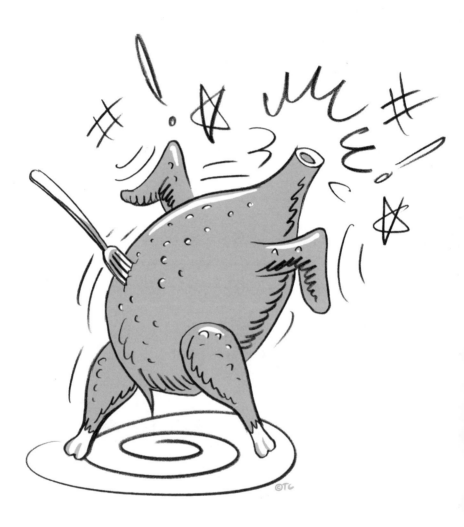

You win! Way to go! You beat Poultry Man.

If you think this way, you have already won. If you are still craving any poultry or you are wondering how you will make it through Thanksgiving without eating any turkey, listen to this statement from Learning Man. "Remember when you cut the cancerous tumors off the chicken? Many of those tumors are not visible on the chicken, so they can't be cut off, and they end up inside your body." How does a cancerous tumor of a dead purple animal that smells like a garbage dump taste? If you decide to keep eating poultry and let Poultry Man beat you, let me know. If you don't want to find out, then you have just won. Congratulations, you did it. Have a Happy Thanksgiving. Go on to your next opponent. You are half way there. Go for it!

"Be kind to animals, don't eat them."

CARNIVORE: Cats, dogs, wolves, bears and other meat-eating animals. They have teeth that are long, sharp, and, pointed, for ripping apart tough raw animal flesh. None of their teeth are flat molar teeth. Their jaws move up and down, not side to side. They drink water with their tongue. Their tongues are rough and thin. They have claws as sharp as knives for ripping flesh. Their stomach is a round sack that secretes 10 to 20 times as much acid as a herbivore. Their intestines are 3 times as long as their trunk. Their intestinal design facilitates rapid expulsion of fleshy matter. Their liver contains enzymes to break down uric acid—at least 10 to 15 times as much uric acid as a herbivore. Their bowels are smooth and short for quick expulsion of waste matter. Their digestive system has the capacity to expel large amounts of foreign cholesterol. Their blood, saliva and urine is very acidic to help break down animal flesh.

HERBIVORE: Horses, pigs, cows, goats and other grass-eating animals. Their front and canine teeth may be sharp or pointed. Their back teeth are flattened for grinding. Their jaw can move both up and down as well as side to side. They drink water by suction. Their tongue is smooth and thick. Their stomach is round and complex which consists of acid 10 to 20 times weaker than a carnivore. Their intestines are at least 8 to 12 times as long as the trunk of their body and are designed for extracting all nutrients from plant fiber. Their liver has a low tolerance for uric acid. Their bowels are sulcified and complex for the reconstitution of waste matter. Their digestive system has no capacity to expel foreign cholesterol. Their saliva is alkaline which contains enzymes to specifically break down starch carbohydrates. Their blood and urine are alkaline. They cool themselves primarily through perspiration. All of their feet are hoofed or they have hands and feet that contain individual digits (fingers and toes) with nails.

FRUGIVORE: Humans and apes. All of their teeth are flat, especially the back molars. They have the dullest canine teeth of all primates. Their jaws move both up and down and side to side. The shape of their face clearly indicates that humans and apes have no ability to rip out entrails with their mouth. They drink water by suction. Their tongue is smooth and thick. Their stomach is round and complex which contains acid that is 10 to 20 times weaker than a carnivore. Their intestines are at least 12 times as long as their trunk, and are an integral part of the most sophisticated juice extractor in the world—the human digestive system. Their liver has a low tolerance for uric acid. Their bowel walls are puckered, convoluted, and full of deep pouches for the reconstitution of waste matter. Their digestive system has no capacity to expel foreign cholesterol. Their saliva is alkaline which contains an enzyme specifically designed to break down starchy carbohydrates. Their blood and urine is alkaline. They cool themselves primarily through perspiration. Their hands and feet contain individual digits with nails and opposable thumbs. Their hands are perfectly designed to reach out, grab fruit and peel it.

(Chart courtesy of Nature's First Law)

Dairy Man

Your next opponent is big bad Dairy Man. Your mother introduced you to him when you were a baby. As far back as you can remember you were told that he was good for you. But you received incorrect information; he is bad for you and will hurt you.

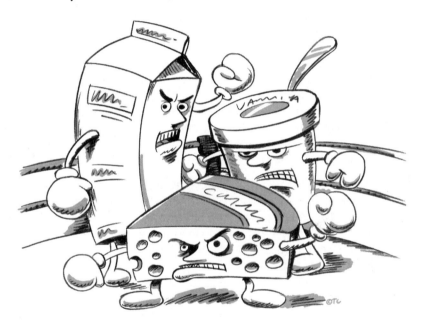

Milk Man, Cheese Man and Ice Cream Man

There are many commercials on television about the benefits of Dairy Man and how he is such an important source of calcium. He tries to use that as one of his punches, but now Learning Man tells you all those commercials are incorrect. Drinking milk actually causes calcium to leach from your bones. Too much animal protein will do that. Milk has excessive amount of animal protein. Although dairy products are promoted as a good source of calcium, as vital for strong bones and as a preventative for osteoporosis, you learned the truth that dairy has been promoted falsely. All dairy products contain significant amounts of saturated fat, allergy inciting cow protein, pesticides, as well as a large load of phosphates, which neutralize the benefits of calcium. Learning Man tells you that the people who make and pay for all those dairy commercials are the same people who sell the products. In fact, dairy is the cause of most diseases in the world today.

Dairy Man has many punches to throw at you. He has his ice-cream punch, his cheese punch, his butter punch, his cake punch and many more. So stay on guard and be aware of them. Once you beat Dairy Man, you will never miss him again.

It is Round One; you and Dairy Man are going blow to blow. Watch out, he throws a butter punch at you. You hit him with a substitute; it is your nut butter punch.

In your corner, between rounds, Learning Man tells you that Dairy Man's products contain a lot of animal protein which can cause allergic reactions in your body. Dairy Man is also extremely mucus-forming, and he could contribute to many different types of inflammation in your body. He wants to hurt you as much as he can and he has the power to do it. Dairy products cause great discomfort to the body. You might not realize this now, but as soon as you defeat him and knock him out of your life forever, you will notice a big difference. Get ready for the next round and beat him. You are on your way towards becoming a champion.

The bell sounds for Round Two and right away Dairy Man charges at you. He throws a cheese punch at you. Now, it is your turn to throw your punch. It is called a seed cheese punch. POW! Seed or nut cheeses are healthier choices that contain no animal products. They are easy to make and taste great. You just soak some seeds or nuts in water for a short period of time. Then you grind them, separating the liquid from the solid by straining through a cheesecloth or sprout bag. It is that simple to make. You just hit Dairy Man with that punch. Way to go!

You are not done yet. Learning Man also tells you that one ounce of cheddar cheese has up to six grams of saturated fat and up to ten milligrams of cholesterol. What a way to finish the round, with two more big punches.

In your corner you are now told that Dairy Man is one of the world's major causes of food poisoning. Salmonella poisoning is the source of most of these cases; listeria is another deadly poison that has been catching up lately. These and other poisons can be deadly if you are not in good health. Chances are that if you are eating dairy products in the first place, you are not in good health. Now you are now really mad and ready to start the next round. You cannot wait to beat Dairy Man.

You throw a punch first this time. When a person ingests any dairy products, they may be digesting many toxic and cancer causing chemicals that were fed to the animals before they were slaughtered. Many toxins are concentrated in the fatty tissues and secretions (such as milk) of these animals.

The next rounds starts. Dairy Man throws a milk punch. Now you throw a punch. It is called your nut milk punch. You hit Dairy Man with a low blow. He didn't want you to learn about nut milks but you trained hard and found out about them. You learned that nut milks are made from nuts such as almonds. The nuts are blended with water and then strained through a cheesecloth or sprout bag. The liquid that is left is the nut milk. You can add sweeteners like bananas, dates or apples to make the milk sweeter. When you make nut milk, you also have nut cheese to use, which was the part you separated from the liquid. Nut Milk is very healthy and it tastes better than any dairy milk that you can buy in the store.

Consuming dairy products does not prevent osteoporosis. If it did, then why are the nations with the highest levels of dairy consumption also the nations with the highest rates of osteoporosis? Now you hit him with your own calcium punch. You say that people can get all the calcium they need from raw fruits and vegetables, especially leafy greens.

All animal byproducts have fat in them. Dairy Man hits the floor. 1-2-3-4-5-6-7-8-9-10. Yes you did it, from this moment on, no more dairy products in your life. Congratulations, you are one step closer to becoming a champion.

With what you have learned, there should be no need for you to desire any dairy products. If you ever run into Craving Man and get any cravings for Dairy Man, just pay a visit to Will Power Man. He will get you through it. Now back to the gym. Time to train for your next opponent.

"My experiences all these years have taught me that more nonsense is spoken about health, diet, symptoms and cures than anything else."

—Morris Krok, Raw food eater for over 50 years

Sugar Man (Sweet he is not)

Your next opponent is Sugar Man. When you beat him, you will be one step closer to your championship. You are so close now you can feel it. You have come a long way and have beat many opponents you thought you could never conquer. This one will not be easy, but you can do it. Sugar Man was once the number one contender. However, there are so many substitutes for Sugar Man today, that he has dropped to number two.

Learning Man says that sugar is the most mobile fighter you will face. He is also very sneaky, has many disguises and he's everywhere. Even where you don't expect to find him, he will show up. Be very careful.

Once you locate him and have him cornered, beating him will be easy. Here are some of his disguises: Brown sugar, honey, syrup, white sugar, caramel, confectioners sugar, lactose and malt. (There are many other forms of sugar under many different names to look out for too. The only way to be sure Sugar Man is not beating you is to avoid eating all processed foods). Those are just the most frequent places that Sugar Man hides. Sometimes not even Learning Man knows where he is. You have to look for him, find him and then do everything in your power to reject him. Make sure Will Power Man is close by your side for this match.

Sugar Man's strategy is to get inside of you and slow you down, to get in your blood and make it sticky like glue. He will try to mess up your insides so much that you will lose the fight with him. He also likes to create dental cavities and destroy your teeth. Most of all, watch out for his deadly knock-out punch. He calls it, "the taste punch." This is what beats most people. Learning to find Sugar Man is one thing, but learning to refuse or reject his taste is another. This is why he is the number two habit to beat. Think positive and you will win. With Willpower Man in your corner, you can't lose. Let's go find and beat Sugar Man.

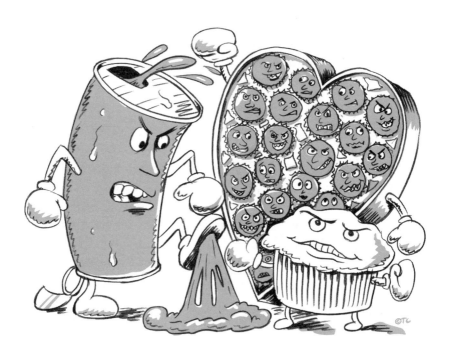

Watch out for the taste punch!

Round One: There he is and you can't wait to hit him and knock him out of your life forever. The bell sounds, where did he go? Look out from behind. He just hit you with a soda punch. Did you know that one can of soda has 39 grams of sugar and that the average American drinks 64 pounds of sugar a year. Ok, so now you will stop drinking soda. Look out! Here comes another punch. Sugar Man is also in processed fruit juices. He just hit you with a commercial fruit juice punch. (Don't get confused, the fruit sugar from raw fruits is not the same as the processed sugar that is added to commercial fruit juices). You didn't even see it coming. You thought that since you stopped drinking soda, this kind of fruit juice would be all right as a substitute. Sugar Man tries to hit you again with another processed fruit juice punch, but you duck. Now you throw a punch—naturally squeezed fruit juice. It is a much better choice. You just hit him and you are one of the few to ever hit Sugar Man. He is surprised and now you are confident. Keep going at him. Don't let up now.

Here comes another punch from Sugar Man. It is called junk food. You see it coming because everyone knows how much sugar is in junk food. Although you see it, you still manage to get hit by it a few times. That is what the junk food punch will do to you. You know it is no good for you, you know it is going to hit you if you don't move, but it tastes so good and is so addicting that you can't help it. Learning Man has some advice for you. You came this far, so if you want to keep going and become a champion, you have to beat Sugar Man. Cookies, cakes, donuts, candy, etc., all of these punches have hit you in the past, but you will not let them hit you anymore.

Now it is time for you to throw some of your own punches. You can make your own natural cookies with dried fruits in a dehydrator. You can make the best tasting natural candies with fruit, and no processed sugar is ever needed. The same goes for cakes and pies. They all taste much better and are healthier for you when you use only natural ingredients. Although they are natural, it is still important not to eat too much of these sweet foods.

I will show you how to make all those great substitutes. We will meet my friend Recipe Man and learn how to keep Sugar Man away from you. First you must beat him. You have him on the ropes and hurt. (Remember when you eat something, even if you read the label and it does not indicate that sugar is there, it can still be present. Maybe it is there under a different name. There are many different types and different forms of sugar, just waiting to hit you and beat you up).

The only way to be sure of what you are eating is to just eat unprocessed fresh organic fruit, vegetables and nuts. Even then, you have to be careful not to overeat even these foods.

When you become a champion, continue to study and learn about everything that might take your title away. If you do, nothing can sneak up on you and beat you. It would be a shame to come this far and lose to Sugar Man. Continue to educate yourself on this topic. Having this information, you just knocked out Sugar Man. Wow, what a great feeling! Just two more opponents to beat and then you are the champion.Go for it!

Giant Grain Man AKA Starch Man

Your next opponent is Giant Grain Man. Be careful, as he is very deceptive. Make sure you work extra hard with Mind Man this time, because Grain Man likes to brainwash people. People are under the impression that they are supposed to eat grains. Mind Man will help you realize this is incorrect.Once you realize this, you will beat Grain Man. Grain Man wants to keep you thinking that he is not only an important, but a necessary part of your diet. Remember what I stated before- *To learn the truth, you must first unlearn all the misinformation you have been taught in the past*. Let's see what Learning Man has to say.

Learning Man tells you that Grain Man should not, as many people believe, be a staple in your diet. In fact, eating grains, especially cooked grains, can kill you. Grain Man's most powerful punch is that he creates a great deal of mucus in the body. He is also difficult to digest. There are many pesticides in grains. He is harmful to the body in an uncooked and sprouted form. When he is cooked, he may be deadly. Let's learn about some of his most famous punches to look out for.

You know about rice and bread, but there are many more grains that you probably haven't heard of. Some of them are millet, amaranth, kamut and quinoa. They can all hurt you if you let them hit you. Rice is the worst grain. It is damaging by itself, but to make it even worse, many processors add deadly food colorings and other additives to make it tastier.

Grain Man knows how to get to people. It is up to you to stop him. You are so close now to becoming a champion. Keep up the good work.

Processed grains include pastas and all flour products, including white bread. You probably know this already and may have switched to whole grain products, thinking that whole grains are much better for you because they are not as processed. Grain Man doesn't want you to know that whole grains can actually be worse for you. This is because a very popular form of whole grain is Grain Man's deadly knockout punch called wheat. Do not underestimate this punch; it will knock you out if you allow wheat to continue hitting you. Let's hear what Learning Man has to say about Grain Man's famous knockout punch.

"Of all the punches that hit you, wheat is certainly the hardest. You will realize this once you start ducking and moving out of the way. The wheat punch is not just an ordinary punch; this punch has something behind it. It is called gluten. Gluten is found in wheat products, and because gluten is unnatural to the human body, everyone is allergic to it. It is very addictive and difficult to stop eating."

"Wheat, barley, rye and oat products all contain gluten. When you eat gluten, it turns to a paste inside your body. This is why it is called gluten—it is actually glue. Just like glue, gluten will stick to the intestinal lining cells in your body and slow you down, leaving you wide open to get hit with all of Grain Man's other punches. Everything you eat that contains gluten will stick to your intestinal wall and form a hard coating as time goes by. This material will, in fact, become so hard and solid that it will be very difficult to get out of your body. Not only does it just sit there, but it also blocks your intestines from receiving nutrients from the food you eat and from distributing them to the rest of the body. The more you are hit with the wheat punch, the more gluten keeps building up inside of you. Some people have five to ten pounds of this waste in their intestines." Wheat can be a deadly punch. Do not let it hit you ever again. If you are hit with it, remember that Willpower Man is in your corner at all times.

If you continue to eat grains in any form, Grain Man will knock you out and you won't even know what hit you. Avoid grains and all grain products. Here are some of Grain Man's punches to watch out for. His white bread, wheat bread, pasta, flour, corn flakes, rice cereal and many other cereal punches; his egg noodle, pancake, waffle, rice, cracker, tortillas, bread roll, bagel, cookies and muffin punches. There are many more punches that Grain Man has. These few are mentioned to give you an example of how many punches he has been hitting you with over the years. Learning Man also tells you about one of Grain Man's deadliest punches—the starch punch—and an even worse one called the cooked starch punch. Starch is in all cooked or sprouted grains and is a poison to the human body. Stay away from it at all costs.

Always think positive; Willpower Man is in your corner at all times. You can beat Grain Man. He will hit you with as many

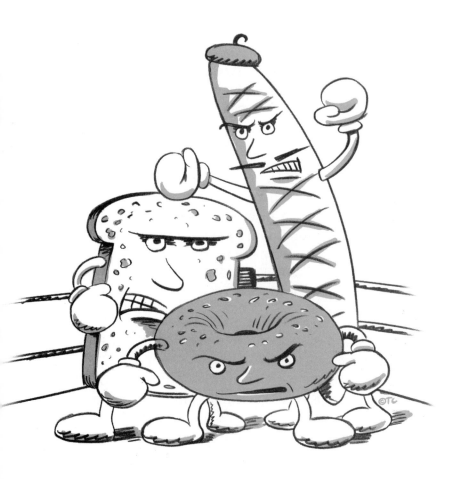

All of these are grains and must be eliminated to become a champion.

punches as you allow. Move out of the way and you will win. There are not too many people that have beaten Grain Man but everyone who has beaten him has gone on to become a champion. This is why he is the number one opponent. Grain Man is very tricky and deceiving. Think positive at all times.

Once you become champion, there will be many other

things to eat. You won't miss any of the poisonous grains. The opponents that you have already beaten will try to stop you from becoming a champion. Dairy Man, Sugar Man, and Egg Man will all join forces with Grain Man to try and beat you. They will tell Grain Man about your weaknesses, and they will form together into candies, cakes and cookies. You have already beaten each of them individually, so why not beat them all together?

You have come this far; you have made a name for yourself and have more support than ever. Nothing can stop you from becoming a champion now, not even Grain Man. Here he comes to the ring. You know so much about him now that he doesn't look so mean any more. In his corner with him are Dairy Man, Egg Man and Sugar Man. Don't even think about them. You already beat them. It is Grain Man that you want to beat now.

The bell sounds to start Round One. You start hitting him and beating him very badly. Dairy Man cannot stand to see it anymore and jumps over the ropes into the ring to help him. You hit Dairy Man with a nut milk punch. Now you turn to Sugar Man who is in Grain Man's corner and you tell him not to even try coming into the ring or you will beat him again.

You turn back to Grain Man, who is hurt. You reach back and with all that you have you hit him with the hardest punch that you have ever thrown. Your support crew is cheering you on. Grain Man is down and out for the count. Dairy Man is also out cold and Sugar Man just ran back to the locker room. 1-2-3-4-5-6-7-8-9-10. Yes, you did it! You beat Grain Man. You feel like you are on top of the world. You are going to fight for the championship. Your corner crew climbs inside the ring to lift you on their shoulders. Everyone is cheering. Nothing can stop you now. You can do anything you want. You are so close to becoming a champion; there's just one more opponent to beat. You can do it! Go for it!

Cooked Food Man Current Champion

This is it! The match that you have worked so hard to get to. Beat Cooked Food Man and you will be a champion. Cooked Food Man will be the hardest of all of the opponents. You have already beaten the others so now you are ready for him. You have knocked out most cooked foods from your life already and there are only a few left. These few are probably the hardest to give up. That is why you needed to train to get to the final match.

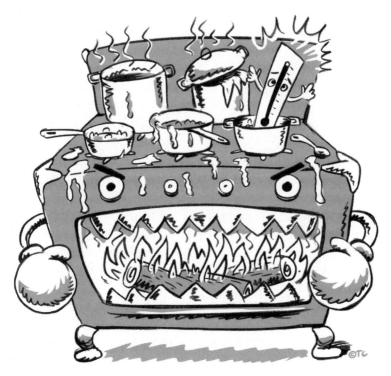

Cooked Food Man. Current champion!

There are foods that you now eat that you may not know are actually cooked. For example, most unshelled nuts and most foods that you see in jars such as applesauce are cooked. Most commercial dried fruit is also cooked. All processed foods are cooked. There are many more foods that might even be labeled "raw" but they are actually cooked. How do you know? The best way to tell if something is cooked or not is to ask yourself if it has been altered. If it is not in its natural form, as originally grown, most likely it is cooked.

I have a friend who thinks that bread isn't cooked because it is cold. This is how some people think. You can only beat what you can fight, which is why it is so important to spend a lot of time with your crew, to learn what you need to win. If you are not sure if something is raw or cooked, don't eat it. If you obtain good quality organic fruits and vegetables, you are getting more than enough nutrients for your body. As for variety, you could eat one fruit every day for the rest of your life and never come close to tasting all the great edible fruits of the world. If you get fresh fruits and vegetables, you will not have to deal with Cooked Food Man ever again.

You must beat Cooked Food Man. If you do not, all the other fights will have been just a waste of time. If you let Cooked Food Man win, you will not just lose the fight, you will lose your life. All cooked food is of no use to the body, but only harms it. As Steve Arlin of Nature's First Law says in his book *The Raw Food Diet*, "*Cooked Food is Poison*." Any food that is cooked is poison. All poisons harm the body and cooked food is no different.

What is wrong with eating poison? Roe Gallo explains it best in her book *Perfect Body*: "*If you eat food that is not completely digestible, it never becomes a nutrient. Since it offers no nutrition to your body, it is processed as toxic waste. The accumulation of waste in your body pollutes it, just as the accumulation of trash pollutes the earth."*

People ask me, "will even just a little cooked food hurt me?" Well, if someone gave you a choice to drink a little poison or a lot of poison, does it matter which you choose? You are still putting poison into your body and any amount of poison will kill you. Cooked Food Man wants to hurt you very badly; in fact, he wants to kill you. Get this into your head. Here's what Dr. John Richter says about cooked food in his book *Nature The Healer:* "*Cooked food has little or no nourishment in it. If you eat it, you are simply starving yourself. Many seem to have the idea that no one can live continuously on raw foods. Raw food is live food, and cooked food is dead food, dead material. When your food is denatured, you eventually denature your whole system; when you put the flesh of cooked vegetables into your stomach, you are truly burying it, as you bury other dead and decaying material in the earth.*"

Learning Man has much to tell you about Cooked Food Man. But remember, before you can learn anything new, you must first clear your head of all the lies that you have been brainwashed into believing.

You notice that you can't seem to find your support crew. They are not totally necessary, but they will make the fight much easier for you to win. Go and find them. Learning Man says to seek out anyone who has beaten Cooked Food Man and ask for advice from these people. Cooked Food Man will have every opponent that you have already beaten cheering him on in order to help him defeat you. There is going to be a funeral one way or the other. Either you kill Cooked Food Man so that he never comes back into your life again, or he beats you. If you lose to him, you will die. It is time to get to work and become a champion. You cannot live a complete life if you are eating cooked food.

Many people will not support you because Cooked Food Man is such a popular champion. Many people are brainwashed and do not want to see him lose. They are used to him always being there. Cooked Food Man has most people thinking that he is their best friend and that he will help them. Cooked Food Man has fooled them all, but he has tricked you for the last time. The other opponents have tried to fool you as well, but you learned that they have been telling you lies. The secret to beating a lie is hearing the truth and believing it. The truth about Cooked Food Man is that he is the opposite of everything you thought he was. He is not your friend, but your enemy; he will not help you, but will hurt you. Cooked food is one of the most unnatural things that you can put into your body.

Life is about living every day, every second, to its fullest. If you eat cooked food, you won't be able to experience this. If you are eating cooked food, you haven't even begun to come close to having that feeling. You will know that feeling when you beat Cooked Food Man and become a champion.

There is no Round One here. If there was a first round, it started when you were born. Cooked Food Man has been kicking your butt everyday, every hour, since then. Every time you ate something cooked, processed or destroyed by heat, you have suffered a punch from Cooked Food Man. When I say destroyed by heat, I don't mean just burned. I mean exactly what I stated, *destroyed*. Listen to what Mind Man tells you. "If you overcook something or burn it, you would throw it away because it does not taste good to you. Cooked Food Man has destroyed it. But, if cooking something for too long will destroy it, then why do people think that cooking something for a short amount of time will not destroy it as well? It surely will."

"The only obvious thing that changes is the taste. The longer something is burned, the worse it will taste. But as soon as it is cooked, no matter for how long, regardless of the taste, it has been destroyed and eventually, it will destroy you." Learning Man tells you the same thing this way: "If you burn something that you are going to eat, it would not taste good to you. It would taste like you are eating ashes. If you don't burn it, it might taste better, but nutritionally it is still the same, as if you were just eating ashes."

Cooked Food Man's most deadly punch is not his timing punch, but his heat punch. This is what will knock you out. Heat is what destroys food. Actually, it destroys all the enzymes in the food. Without enzymes, you could not exist. With inadequate enzymes, you would exist, but not to your fullest capacity. You would live with diseases and sicknesses, like most people do today. When you digest cooked food, you lose many important and valuable enzymes.

Don't heat it and you will be able to eat it!

Most people have been digesting cooked foods since they were born. We eat cooked food before we can walk or talk. If you don't stop eating cooked food soon, it will be much harder for you to beat Cooked Food Man in the future. Now is a good time to visit Change Man. If you can't beat Cooked Food Man now, what makes you think that you will beat him in the future? You have made many changes already, one more and you will be a champion.

When you eat natural foods, you preserve important enzymes. This is one of the secrets to a healthy life and it is a reason why you must beat Cooked Food Man. When you do beat him and clean out your body, physical discomfort in your body will vanish and remain absent unless you let new opponents beat you. Then and only then, will you know what true health really feels like. It will not be easy, but it will be well worth it.

Cooked Food Man will try to beat you with his cravings punch. He will do anything he can to defeat you; he is poison. You have already knocked out all the other bad habits that you thought you could never live without, and you are starting to feel true health again. No need to stop now. Don't be fooled by Cooked Food Man. If something is cold, that doesn't mean it hasn't been cooked. Most processed foods have been cooked, so to play it safe, stay away from all processed food.

If you still are not convinced that Cooked Food Man will kill you with his heat punch, boil a pot of water and then stick your finger into it. Does it hurt? Well, what do you think happens to the food that you put into that water?

Let's look at another way of describing what cooked food does to you. Remember the popular television commercial about drugs? The ad would show an egg being cracked into the frying pan. The announcer would say: *this is your brain on drugs.* Then they would show the egg being fried in the frying pan. Just change the last line in that commercial from *this is your brain on drugs* to *this is your body on cooked food.*

Once you learn the truth about health, you will become a champion. You have to knockout Cooked Food Man for the last time and never look back. ***To become a champion, you have to unlearn the lies that you have been taught about cooked food.***

LIES

-Cooked food is important.

-Cooked food makes digestion easier on your body.

-Cooked food has many vitamins and minerals.

-Cooked food will give you energy.

-Cooked foods get fully digested and leave the body in a few hours.

-We could not live without cooked foods.

-If you continue to eat a cooked food diet, you will live a long and healthy life.

-Eating cooked foods will protect you from becoming sick.

TRUTHS

-Cooking food destroys the digestive enzymes in food. This forces your body to work harder at digestion.

-Heat destroys vitamins and minerals in food, as well as killing enzymes.

-Cooked food will drain your energy.

-If you continue to eat a cooked food diet, you will get diseases and live an unhealthy, unhappy life.

-Cooked food causes constipation and remains in the intestines for days, weeks and sometimes, even years.

-You cannot live life to its fullest when you eat cooked foods.

-Cooked foods are unnatural.

Cooked food is dead food. If you eat dead food you will have dead reactions. For an example, take fresh, raw spinach. It is crispy and tastes nice and fresh. You hear that nice crisp sound with every bite. It is alive. Now put that spinach into a pot of boiling water and cook it for one minute or less. The spinach is now soft and dull, lacking flavor, nutrients, vitamins and enzymes. You killed the spinach; it is now dead. If you eat that spinach, Cooked Food Man will kill you. This happens to so many people everyday. Why must people cook their foods? The point is plain and simple to understand: ***Eat a 100% raw-food diet and you will live your life to the fullest!*** If you cannot eat something in its raw form, do not eat it at all.

For another example, look at any animals in the wild. They don't eat cooked food. They never do. Humans are the only species that cooks their food. All other species eat food the way it was intended, in its most natural raw state, unless humans feed them unnatural cooked food. Because they do not eat cooked food, animals in the wild do not get toxemia (diseases) as humans do.

Animals experience much more stress than humans. Stress for us is losing our jobs or not having money. For wild animals, stress is losing their life. They constantly have to watch their backs. If they do not remain aware of their surroundings all the time, larger animals might eat them. Still, with all the stress they experience, they have no toxemia (diseases) among them. Compare that to house pets like cats and dogs, who are fed cooked and processed foods. Most house pets get one kind of toxemia (disease) or another, the same way humans do. This is because they eat the same food humans do. That is why veterinarians tell you not to feed your house pet food from the table; it is not good for them, it will make them sick. Well, if it will make your pet sick, why wouldn't it make you sick too?

Beating Cooked Food Man will not be easy. The older you are, the harder he will be to defeat. This is because you have been beaten up for so many years. Do not let Cooked Food Man hit you anymore. Start throwing some punches of your own. Your corner crew will help you.

In the following chapters, you will learn what to eat and how to eat, in order to defeat Cooked Food Man and become a champion. I will give you all the information you will need to eliminate all cooked food from your life. I will explain to you how to do it in stages, in order to make the transition as smooth as possible. If you want to beat Cooked Food Man, this is your opportunity to do so.

Once you finish this book, you will have all the knowledge you need! If you continue to eat cooked food, Cooked Food Man will eventually kill you. Do you want him to always beat you up just a little or not at all? If you leave any room open for him, you never know when he will hurt you. If you let him beat you a little, he will always know how to defeat you. You will never be a true champion. You must get him out of your life completely, not just partially. You can get close to being a champion, but it is not the same. You do not want to be anything less than the best. You must give up all cooked food to become the best. Incomplete efforts produce incomplete results.

You are now educated about Cooked Food Man. You know how damaging all cooked food is for you. You know it will kill you if you continue to eat it. It will make your life a living hell, filled with sickness and disease, until he finally does kill you. Now is the time to decide to become a champion or to throw out of the window all your hard work up to this point. You are standing in the ring with Cooked Food Man. Are you going to let him continue to beat you up and to kill you, or are you going to knock him out and become champion?

Your body is an amazing work of art. Physically, it can take much abuse. If you eat a little cooked food, your body will be able to deal with it for a certain amount of time. However, little by little, this food will take its toll on your body until it kills you.

If the food you eat has no value and cannot supply your body with what it needs, you are actually starving yourself and, in time, you will starve to death. If everyone ate a 100% cooked food diet for a period of time, they would all die of starvation, because cooked food has nothing the body can use. It is dead. You cannot survive on eating ashes, and cooked food is just good tasting ashes.

No one eats a 100% cooked food diet. Even the average person eating the "Standard American Diet" (the SAD diet) eats some raw food. For example, if someone eats a hamburger with lettuce and tomatoes, he is consuming very little raw food, but he is eating some. While the hamburger is killing them, the small amount of raw food is keeping them from starving.

This is proof of the power and vitality of raw foods. It helps cooked food eaters survive. It makes raw food eaters thrive. In essence, we are all raw food eaters; some of us just eat some cooked food too.

Because cooked food is so addictive, it will be harder to restrict yourself to small amounts of it than none at all. This is why a 100% raw-food diet is the only answer! Even if your diet consists of 99.9% raw foods, it will be too difficult to maintain. That 0.1 percent of cooked food will keep the taste for and the addiction to cooked food in your body. Consuming 100% raw foods will cause you to lose the cravings and the taste for Cooked Food Man. Any amount less than 100% will not do it. Cooked Food Man wants you to continue eating at least a little cooked food, so you never lose the taste for it and the addiction to it. If you eat any amount of cooked food you will always crave more. You will never lose the taste for it and that is when Cooked Food Man will beat you. The only way to lose the taste and to avoid the cravings is to knockout Cooked Food Man completely. Eat no more cooked food, and you will thrive.

The longer you wait, the harder it will be. If you choose to knockout Cooked Food Man and live, congratulations, you are a champion in the making. Your corner crew will help you get there. In the next chapter, you will learn how to do it. Your corner crew will tell you what to eat and how to eat it. They will also tell you about all the new opponents that will try to challenge you and they will train you to defeat them as well.

Like every new champion, you will have to adopt a new name when you knockout Cooked Food Man and stop eating cooked food. We will call you Raw Food Man or Raw Food Woman. You are going to kill Cooked Food Man before he kills you. Congratulations. You made the right choice! You know why you must beat Cooked Food Man. Now go and get the information you need to do it!

"In society people are put into situations where they feel they have to eat, even if they're not hungry. For example, people always eat when on a plane or at the movies. They are not only addicted to the food, but they are addicted to society's crazy concepts as well."

—Paul Nison

"Why do people cook their vegetables and not their fruits? Because society says so, that's why. People should question that. It is okay and normal to eat our fruits raw, but to eat anything else raw is not normal? We should stop listening to society and start listening to our bodies!"

—Paul Nison

"Any food that needs to be heated to make them palatable or to destroy toxic poisons in that food, shows that they are not natural foods in the first place."

—Morris Krok

It is a good idea, when you become a champion, to keep a journal of your progress and the changes that your body goes through. Your body will go through many changes and it will always be useful to look back and reflect on where you started out and how far you have come.

4 | RAW DIET:
What can you eat and when can you eat it

To beat Cooked Food Man you must eliminate all cooked food from your diet. As you progress towards this goal, you will notice many changes in your health. Some of them may seem like negative changes at first, but in reality, only positive changes will be taking place. Stay focused and you will get past these changes. Your goal is to restrict your eating to only raw fruits, vegetables, nuts and seeds.

If you decided not to make the transition in stages, you will not have to read parts of this chapter. If you are able to change from a cooked food diet to a raw food diet overnight, congratulations. You beat Cooked Food Man and you are now the champion. If you decided to make the change systematically in stages, I will now tell you how.

Phase One

One way to accomplish the shift that I recommend is to eat only fruit until noon everyday. (I am assuming most people reading this work the typical 9 to 5 workday. If you work a different shift or work nights, just eat fruit for the first five hours after you wake up). When you do this, you will feel hungry at first because, like most people, you are used to eating a heavy breakfast in the morning. Don't worry; after continuing this pattern for a while, your body will adapt to it. You will see how much more energy you have, without drinking coffee or eating a heavy breakfast.

Consider this "fruit to noon" a part of your punch combination that will knockout Cooked Food Man. Continue to skip breakfast if that is already your habit. There is nothing wrong with not eating breakfast, but if you are skipping breakfast, be careful. Make sure you are not drinking coffee, or having anything else as your breakfast. This meal should consist of just fruit or nothing at all. ***No unnatural foods or unnatural drinks before noon in Phase 1.*** If you must drink something, have water or fresh-squeezed fruit juice. By fresh, I don't mean commercial juice. If it is commercial, it is processed and not truly natural. A hand citrus juicer cost under $20 and is very easy to use.

For most people, the average amount of time spent in Phase 1 will be about a month, enough time to get adjusted to this new style of eating. The shorter this period is, the better. If you have a hard time adjusting, seek out your support crew and get advice. People who have "been there" and "gone through it" can be a tremendous help. You might not initially be aware of their existence, but the more you get into the raw food lifestyle, the more they will appear. When you are comfortable with Phase 1, move on to Phase II.

Phase Two

Now that you feel comfortable eating nothing at all or just fruit until noon on a daily basis, proceed to Phase II. The final goal is to eat 100% raw food every day. This is the only way you can beat Cooked Food Man and become the champion. If you are eating any amount less than 100% raw foods, you are not on a raw food diet. You are just eating a lot of raw food and you are still fighting Cooked Food Man.

There are two ways you can handle Phase II. The first is to expand the hours of your fruit eating from up till noon to until 3 PM. That's only three more hours. Once you are comfortable with that, extend the period to 4 PM, then 5 PM and so on. After noon, you can add leafy green vegetables and nuts to your fruit diet. Before you know it, you will knockout Cooked Food Man and be eating 100% raw foods.

The second way is to keep on eating fruit, up to noon every day and then, during the middle of the day, eat whatever you choose. Later, for an evening meal, go back to just eating fruit again, along with leafy green vegetables and nuts. When you get used to that, you can slowly but surely fill the gap with raw foods until you knockout Cooked Food Man completely. Then you become the champion.

"Some people live to eat, but we should eat to live."

Raw Food Diets

There are many different styles of the raw food diet. Fruitarian, live foods and Natural Hygiene diets are just a few of them. (See dictionary in the back of this book for different types of raw food diets). I would highly recommend the Natural Hygiene diet, with a few adjustments, as the best style of them all. Study all of the different raw diets and decide which is best for you. Whichever one you choose, make sure the food you eat is of the best quality possible. This would mean both organic and fully ripened. "Don't Ever Panic, Just Eat Organic" and do not overeat.

113

"You can't always control what you breathe, what touches your skin or what you see. And you don't have complete control over what goes into your mind. But you do have total control over what you put into your mouth. Your health and longevity depends primarily on what you eat. What you eat determines mainly whether your body is healthy or diseased. Simple and absolute."

—Roe Gallo From her book *Perfect Body*

> It's not only about what you eat. It all starts
> with what you don't eat.

Food Combining

Food Combining Man is a very important part of your team. There are many different types of raw foods, and different types will take different amounts of time to digest. Your body will have to work harder to digest foods if you eat them in poor combinations. You want your body to waste as little energy as possible. For this reason, it is important to combine your food properly. There are many books written about food combining. I suggest you read some of them to learn as much as you can about food combining. (Refer to the recommended reading list in the back of this book). I have also added a food combining chart to help you in following the rules of food combining for best digestion. To help you understand appropriate food combining combinations and to make it simpler for you, always remember to eat liquid foods with other liquid foods, and more dense foods with other dense foods.

The best foods for the human body are ripe, organic fruits and vegetables. The best fruits and vegetables for the human body will contain the highest water content possible. A good way to measure water content is to put any food through a juicer. The more liquid that comes out, the higher the water content of that food and the more beneficial that food is for you. Picture your body as a juicer. If eaten in its raw state, there will be no better choice as food for the human body.

Cooking will evaporate most of the water and make the perfect food dense, dull, and dead. That's only part of what makes it so bad. Try putting a piece of bread in a juicer and you will see the juicer work very hard, but still nothing will come out. If you continue, eventually the juicer will break, just as your body will get diseased if you continue to eat cooked foods.

When you eat one food as your entire meal (a mono-diet), you do not have to think about food combining. However, if you are going to eat many different kinds of food in the same meal, you should study and follow the rules of food combining. The following chart will inform you about food combining.

Make sure you chew every bite of food about 30 times, until it becomes liquid. You want to mix your saliva with the food. Good digestion starts in the mouth. Remember your stomach does not have teeth. "Chew your drinks and drink your meals."

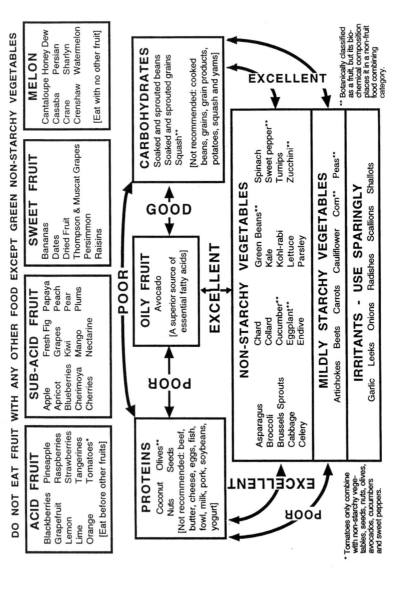

FOOD COMBINING CHART

DO NOT EAT FRUIT WITH ANY OTHER FOOD EXCEPT GREEN NON-STARCHY VEGETABLES

ACID FRUIT

Blackberries Pineapple
Grapefruit Raspberries
Lemon Strawberries
Lime Tangerines
Orange Tomatoes*

[Eat before other fruits]

SUB-ACID FRUIT

Apple Fresh Fig Papaya
Apricot Grapes Peach
Blueberries Kiwi Pear
Cherimoya Mango Plums
Cherries Nectarine

SWEET FRUIT

Bananas
Dates
Dried Fruit
Thompson & Muscat Grapes
Persimmon
Raisins

MELON

Cantaloupe Honey Dew
Casaba Persian
Crane Sharlyn
Crenshaw Watermelon

[Eat with no other fruit]

CARBOHYDRATES

Soaked and sprouted beans
Soaked and sprouted grains
Squash**

[Not recommended: cooked beans, grains, grain products, potatoes, squash and yams]

OILY FRUIT

Avocado

[A superior source of essential fatty acids]

PROTEINS

Coconut Olives** Seeds
Nuts

[Not recommended: beef, butter, cheese, eggs, fish, fowl, milk, pork, soybeans, yogurt]

NON-STARCHY VEGETABLES

Asparagus Chard Green Beans** Spinach
Broccoli Collard Kale Sweet pepper**
Brussels Sprouts Cucumber** Kohl-rabi Turnips
Cabbage Eggplant** Lettuce Zucchini**
Celery Endive Parsley

MILDLY STARCHY VEGETABLES

Artichokes Beets Carrots Cauliflower Corn** Peas**

IRRITANTS - USE SPARINGLY

Garlic Leeks Onions Radishes Scallions Shallots

EXCELLENT

GOOD

POOR

POOR

EXCELLENT

EXCELLENT

POOR

* Tomatoes only combine with non-starchy vegetables, seeds, nuts, olives, avocados, cucumbers and sweet peppers.

** Botanically classified as a fruit, but its bio-chemical composition places it in a non-fruit food combining category.

Chart by David Klein

116

Raw Food Pearamid

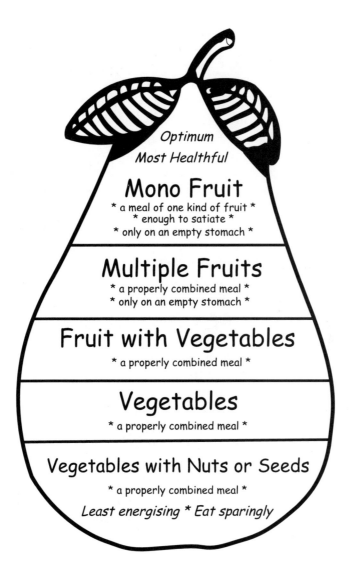

Optimum
Most Healthful

Mono Fruit
* a meal of one kind of fruit *
* enough to satiate *
* only on an empty stomach *

Multiple Fruits
* a properly combined meal *
* only on an empty stomach *

Fruit with Vegetables
* a properly combined meal *

Vegetables
* a properly combined meal *

Vegetables with Nuts or Seeds
* a properly combined meal *
*Least energising * Eat sparingly*

Chart by David Klein

The best time to eat and how often you should eat.

A common question people ask me is "what is the best time to eat and how often should one eat?"

An important point to remember here is never to eat by the clock; you should eat to satisfy your hunger. Instead of thinking what time you should eat, it is more important to think about what time you shouldn't eat. Everyone overeats, and if they ate less often, they would have much better health to show for it. To answer this question, read what Vera Ricther, in Mrs. Richter's *COOK-Less Book*, has to say:

"Eat only when absolutely hungry. Always work for several hours before partaking of food. The secret of health is not only moderation but occasional abstinence. As soon as we become inclined to use stimulants or condiments to relish our food, it is high time to give our digestive organs a rest."

You have been trained to eat breakfast when you wake up, to eat lunch in the afternoon around noon, and to eat dinner in the evening at about 6 PM. If you've ever thought about this, you would realize that it does not make any sense. Get the idea out of your head that you have to eat at a certain time. If it is noon, and you are not hungry, it is okay to skip lunch.

To help you get out of the habit of eating meals at a certain time, don't label your meal as "breakfast," "lunch," or "dinner." There is no such thing as lunch or dinner. When you are not eating, you are abstaining from food, you are fasting. Therefore, when you do eat, you are breaking that fast. Then, you are eating breakfast (break-fast). So the only meal you ever eat, no matter what time, is breakfast.

Eat when you feel hungry, when your body tells you it needs food. ***It is important to learn the difference be-***

tween hunger and a false appetite. Most people have never felt true hunger. Your body can thrive without food for weeks, even months. If you skip a meal or two, or don't eat for a day or two, you are not going to starve to death.

Since the body can last for weeks without food, it is very rare for anyone to reach the point of true hunger. This brings us to the question: If one doesn't reach true hunger, how does he or she know when it is time to eat? The answer is to eat when you feel you need food for its value, and not because of the clock or for emotional reasons.

Once you are eating, how do you know when you have had enough? How much food should be eaten to remain in the best of health? The best answer to these questions is in *The Natural Food For Man* by Hereward Carrington, who was a great champion of raw food eating who lived in the early 1900's. He states:

"Every individual should restrict himself to the smallest quantity that he finds, from careful investigation and experiment, will meet the wants of his system, knowing that whatever is more than this is harmful."

Before eating, ask yourself, "do you need to eat, or do you want to eat?" If the former, enjoy your meal. Follow correct food combining rules. Do not overeat. If the latter, it is not the right time to eat. When you do eat, stop eating when you feel like you have had enough—when you feel full, but not too full. Do not overeat just because there is food left to be eaten. If you are full, you do not have to finish it.

Food is a bad habit, and force of habit is why most people eat most of the time. The body has little use for food. Fresh clean air is what nourishes the body, not food. As Doctor Hilton

Hotema states in his book *Man's Higher Consciousness;* *"The body cells do not depend on what man eats. The cells are far above the nutritional level, are independent of nutrition, and are self-existent and eternal. Food cannot sustain what it cannot produce. As the body is not the product of food, it is actually not sustained by food. If the cells of the body depend on food, man should continue to grow and live as long as he had sufficient food."*

If the body depended on food to survive, there would be no such thing as death by natural causes. In fact, there would be no death at all, other than through physical accidents, and man would live for hundreds of years. Dr. Hotema goes on to say: *"What food does not produce, it cannot sustain. As the body is not composed of extraneous material, we cannot feed it with such material, as such material is foreign to its constitution. In the attempt to nourish cells, which need no nourishment, lies one of the errors that hurries man to the grave. Feeding increases the degenerative process, whereas fasting, the opposite course, institutes the opposite effect-the process of rejuvenation."*

After your body has fully adjusted to a more natural way of eating, you will feel the need for food very infrequently. Your final goal is for your body to get a feeling of fullness on the smallest amounts of the highest quality raw foods and nothing else. There is a saying *"to lengthen thy life, lessen thy meals."* You will be able to do this once your body is used to 100% raw foods. As Resting Man told you, rest the insides of your body as well as the outside. *Eat as little as needed to feel good*. Many people today eat too much food, much more than their bodies require. They are eating themselves to death. It can be easy to overeat, especially when the foods taste good.

Certain people will require more food than others will. It depends upon your degree of physical activity. A professional athlete will need more food than an office worker who never exercises. As long as you listen to your body, you will know how much food you need.

People overeat for many reasons. The main one is to satisfy emotions, not to satisfy hunger. This is why you should never eat if you have any stress or you are not at total peace with yourself. ***Eating while you are angry, anxious, fearful, tired or upset will lead to overeating.*** Knowing when to eat, when not to eat and how to eat is very important. When you eat, don't hurry or eat too fast, and make sure you chew your food until it becomes a liquid. If your are drinking, swirl it in your mouth to mix it with saliva before swallowing.

Another reason for overeating is that food tastes too good to stop eating. This can't happen when your meal only consists of one food. This is a mono diet. Your body will tell you when to stop eating on a mono diet of good quality raw food. The food will stop tasting good to you once you are full. This is nature's way of making sure you don't overeat.

"The kitchen table will entice you to overeat. Just because people have a table, they feel they have to get the best use out of it. Get rid of your table and it will help you to avoid overeating."

Another reason people overeat is peer pressure. Some people will go out to eat with their friends, and just because their friends are eating something, they will also eat, although they are not hungry. Be careful with this type of situation.

Whatever the reason you do overeat, be aware of your thoughts and what is happening when you eat. Take notes if you must, and learn from your mistakes and weaknesses. Also, don't talk when you eat. Concentrate on the food. If you observe any animal, you will never see them vocalize with food in their mouth. How bizarre it would be to see a dog trying to bark with food in his mouth. You will never see that.

If food is overeaten or the food combining rules are not followed, the food you eat will not be digested properly and this will lead to many problems, including toxemia. Dr. Carrington explains in *Fasting For Health And Long Life*:

"When food is not properly digested, it causes trouble! An excess of protein results in putrefaction; an excess of carbohydrates, in fermentation. Both are bad; both result in unpleasant and ultimately serious symptoms. Gases and poisons are formed within the body, which pass into the blood-stream and affect the tissues and organs, and even the delicate nerve-cells of the brain. The mental and emotional life are affected, no less than the grosser physical elements. Waste material accumulates, toxins are formed, which poison and block the tiny blood vessels. The body becomes choked with the excess. Desperately, nature tries to get rid of this load by driving the eliminating organs to greater and greater efforts, until they break down under the strain. When this occurs, the patient is already in the throes of illness. He is now a really sick man."

What makes Dr. Carrington's remark so scary is that most people overeat. This is why there is so much disease (toxemia) in the world. I guarantee if everyone ate less than half of the food they now consume, all diseases rates would decline precipitously. Anyone who knows about true health will realize this. People are killing themselves with food. As the great health writer Arnold Ehret states in all his books, *"Life is the tragedy of nutrition."*

***"More deaths happen in the kitchen than in any
other room in the house."***

—Morris Krok

It is very easy to overeat on any type of food, raw or cooked. On the contrary, it is almost impossible to undereat, if a person is eating the highest quality raw foods. People should stop worrying about not eating enough food, as so many tend to do, and start realizing that they're eating to excess. It is more important to eat small amounts of good quality food than to overeat on any kind of food.

From a physiological point of view, a person can live sixty days or more on clean water and air without any food. This shows how much most people overeat. The average person eats three meals a day, with snacking meals in between those main meals, adding up to five meals per day. Multiply that by sixty, the number of days a person can live without food, and you get 300. A person is putting 300 meals into his body that his body doesn't need. Even if you are not fasting and, let's say, eating two meals a day, that would add up to 120 meals in those 60 days. This would mean that, in just two months time, the average person is eating 180 meals more than they should be eating.

To make matters worse, of the 180 to 300 meals a person overeats, most, if not all of them, are of no use to the body because they are not good quality meals. It is like putting a lot of bread into the gas tank of a car with very little gas. The car will run on that small amount of gas for a while until all the bread clogs it up, and then it will no longer be able to run.

As Dr. Carrington said, putting more food in your body than it needs will make you a very sick person. This is why the average person gets sick. Generally, you are considered very lucky if you do not get any diseases in your lifetime, yet actually, there is no luck involved here. It is common sense; if you overeat, you cannot be a champion.

> Do not eat when you are angry, anxious, fearful, upset, or tired.

Snacks throughout the day

I do not recommend snacking throughout the day after you have been on the raw diet for some time. But when starting out, during your transition to a raw food diet, it is okay as long as the snacks are raw and you follow correct food combining rules and stop eating when you are full. Snack on any fruits, nuts, or raw candies as you feel you need to, and no more. In time you will lose the desire to snack throughout the day. Listen to your body and you will know when you are ready to take your diet to the next level. Remember, don't name your meals. When you snack, you are still eating a meal (breakfast). You want to get to the point where you are eating no more than two meals per day (unless you are doing a lot of physical work).

Recipes

You can make many great tasting recipes with raw foods. Some people might have trouble adjusting at first to just eating mostly fruits and leafy green salads. To help make the process easier, I have included a few raw recipes. Recipe Man will help you learn about making raw recipes. In addition, in the back of this book is a listing of some good recipe books that will help you. In the beginning, you will enjoy these great tasting recipes and you may want to incorporate them into your diet. As time goes by, and you gravitate to eating more of a mono diet, you will only feel the need to consume these meals sparingly.

When I was eating foods that were unnatural, there were many great tasting fruits and vegetables that I didn't like. As my tastebuds became clean again, I began to love those same fruits and vegetables I didn't like before. Don't ever give up on nature.

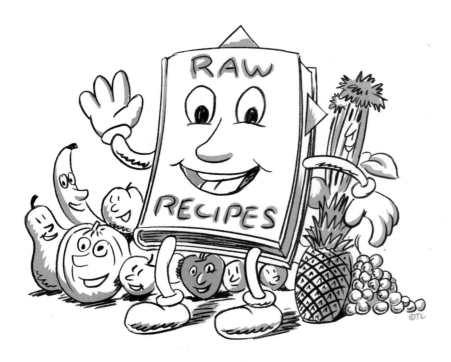

Recipe Man will give you many great recipes to make and enjoy.

125

Recipe Man says that when people start a raw-food diet, they want to experience the fullness that cooked foods gave them. Here are a few good recipes that will help you feel that same fullness. These recipes are okay to eat during a transition to a raw-food diet. Once you are on a 100% raw-food diet, only eat these recipes sparingly, if at all. It is always best to eat a mono diet. If you must eat these or any recipes, follow the food combining chart as closely as possible. Eating without following proper food combining guidelines or overeating, even if it is all raw foods, will give you indigestion and gas, will zap your energy levels and lead to toxemia.

Next, follow the food combining guidelines as closely as possible. Eat sweet fruits with sweet fruits, citrus fruits with citrus fruits, and low moisture fruits with more low moisture fruits. Always eat melons by themselves, with no other fruit. Melons do not digest well with other fruits as their digestion times are much quicker than other foods, including fruits.

It is okay to eat these recipes every now and then at first, but ideally, you want to eat as close to nature as possible. This would mean eating one food at a time, a mono diet.

The more time you stay on the raw diet, the more your body will get used to a mono diet (a meal of only one kind of food) and you will not need to mix foods in combinations. Everyone's body is different, and getting to the level of the mono diet will take varying amounts of time for people. Some will be ready for it much sooner than others. It can take weeks, months or even years. As long as you understand why you must eat this way, you eventually will be ready to do so. Your body has to be ready for the changes, and so does your mind.

Enjoy these delicious recipes. They are easy to make and

taste great. There are also many raw food recipe books available today. Check the recommended reading section in the back of this book for some of them.

Recipes

Soups & Dressings

Basic Raw Dressing

4 oz of Tahini
1/2 Lemon, Juiced
1 Clove Garlic
Pinch of Cayenne Pepper
1 tbs. of Dulse, Kelp or Namo Shoyu

Blend and serve.

Tomato Basil Dressing

2 Tomatoes
1 Garlic Clove
1/2 Lemon, Juiced
Handful of Basil

Blend or put in food processer

Tahini Raisin Dressing

1/2 Cup Raisins, soaked
2 tbs. Tahini
1/2 Lemon, juiced

2 tbs. Onion
1/2 cup water

Blend and serve.

Raw tomato Soup

3 Tomatoes
1 Clove Garlic
1 tbs. Onion
1 tbs. Parsley
1 tbs. Basil
1/2 Lemon, juiced

Blend and serve

You can make many different raw dressings and soups. The trick is just to put any fruits, vegetables, nuts or seeds into a blender and blend them all together. Add water as needed for consistency; after that, adjust to your taste. Example: if you make a dressing in which that you want more zing, just add lemon juice. There are many great raw recipe books, buy one or two. At first, prepare the recipes as indicated, then add anything else you want to adjust the taste to your liking.

Entrees

Raw Mushroom Pizza Pie

1 Portabello Mushroom
1 Tomato
1 Lemon, juiced
Any nut or seed spread (almond butter, tahini, etc.). Stem

and clean mushroom cap. Then turn cap upside down like a plate. Squeeze lemon juice over cap. Next, put nut spread over the cap. Slice the tomato and place slices over the spread. Enjoy! (If you want, you can add avocado slices, olives or anything else that you might like)

Raw Pasta with Sauce

Zucchini Primavera
Pasta
Shred Zucchini in saladacco (food processor)
Sauce for pasta
2 Big Tomatoes
Handful Sun-Dried Tomatoes
2 Cloves Garlic
1 Handful Basil
1/2 Handful Fresh Oregano
1/4 Onion
1/2 Lemon, juiced

Blend all ingredients

Veggies you may add on top: Broccoli, Cauliflower, Zucchini, Squash, Mushrooms, and Sun-dried tomatoes.

Carrots and Sweet Potato Salad

Shredded Carrots & Sweet Potato
Raisins (soaked 5 min. in water)
Tahini
Pine nuts

Use as much of each as you like.
Mix in a big bowl and serve

Tomato Sauce

6 Tomatoes
Handful of sun-dried tomatoes, soaked
Basil to taste
Oregano to taste
6 Garlic Cloves
Zucchini pieces

Blend and serve.

Desserts

Basic Raw Fruit Pie

For the crust: 2 to 4 cups nuts (any kind) and 6 to 15 dates. Blend in a food processor. Do not add any water. After blending, put mixture into a 9-inch pie plate. Flatten it out with your hands. Optional: You can add shredded coconut or carob powder to give the crust a different flavor.

For the filling: Mix the meat of 3 baby coconuts in a blender with 1/2 cup of coconut water. Add 1 teaspoon psyllium seed husk powder to thicken the liquid (buy it in any health food store). Next slice up any fruit and place it at the bottom of the piecrust. (I like bananas best) Then pour some of the liquid over the sliced fruit. Then place another layer of different fruits .After pie is in shell, sprinkle some shredded coconut over the liquid and decorate with raisins or nuts. Be creative. Enjoy.

Basic Raw Pie Crust

Pecans, Walnuts, Dates, Cinnamon,
4 cups nuts 1 cup dates

Mix all in a food processor and press with your
hand in to a glass pie plate

Coconut Fruit Pie Filling

1/2 Cup Coconut water of Baby Coconuts
Coconut meat of 3 Baby coconuts
2 Bananas Sliced
1/2 Tsp. Psyllium Seed Powder
Top with fruit of choice

Carob Pie Filling or chocolate pudding

Meat of 1 Baby Coconut
1 Handful Pine Nuts
1 Apple, peeled
1 cup Dates
1/2 cup Water
Carob powder to taste
2 spoons psyllium husk

Blend.

Strawberry Pie Filling

Same as for Coconut Fruit Pie, Just add 2 handfuls of
Strawberries and 4 dates to the coconut meat filling

Parfait
2 Cups Walnuts
10 Dates
1 1/2 Cups Water
1 tbs. Vanilla or Walnut Extract
Sprinkle with nutmeg

Blend

Brownies

1 Cup Pine nuts
1 Cup Sunflower Seeds
Opt. 1 tsp. of Vanilla

Process and mix nuts together
Blend 1 Banana and 6 Dates with water
Add 1/2 cup carob powder

Mix nuts and fruit together and dehydrate 24 hours.

Date Balls

Roll 1 date into a ball. Place a pecan or almond in the
middle, then roll in coconut or in sesame seeds.

Pudding

1 cup coconut water
4 dates
1 cup pine nuts
Grated nutmeg to garnish

Carob Truffles

Walnuts
Carob powder
Water

Blend and roll in coconut or sesame seeds.

Crackers

Carrot Pulp, 1 Cup
Sunflower seeds, 1 Cup
Sesame seeds, 1 Cup (1/2 in mix; 1/2 on top when done)
1 small Red onion
1/4 cup or less of Lemon juice
Optional: add Garlic, olive oil, 1 tsp. curry, 1 tsp. Cumin,

Dehydrate 3 hours on teflex sheet, remove sheet, then
dehydrate 4 more hours

Drinks

Coconut shake
Meat of one coconut
1/2 cup coconut water.

Blend and serve

Nut Milk

1 Cup Almonds (or other nuts)
2 cups water
Blend and strain
Add
1 Banana or 1 apple
1 Cup Dates

Blend

Recap

* Plan your meals wisely, listen to your body.

* Mono diet is best, followed by a fruit diet along with correct food combining rules.

* Choose organic over non-organic whenever possible.

* Eat foods in their most natural form, raw and unprocessed.

* Learn what true hunger is and eat only when true hunger is present.

* Do not dwell on the opponents that you have already beaten.

Some people say raw foods are not for everybody or raw foods don't agree with them. Raw foods are for anyone who wants to live without discomfort, sickness and disease. If you think that raw foods do not agree with you, it is you that does not agree with raw foods. This is the way we were meant to eat. This is the first law of nature. Open your mind and re-examine everything. Let raw foods agree with you and you will see the benefits. You will become a champion.

I have a friend who works for a very popular orange juice company. He was at my house and was squeezing oranges for juice. I asked him why didn't he just drink the orange juice that his company makes. He told me he would never drink any commercial orange juice or any other kind of commercial fruit juice. I asked him why. He told me when they collect the oranges to be juiced, it is bad enough that the oranges are not washed, but they put all of the dirty oranges into a huge compressor and squeeze them all together to squeeze out the juice. Right before they squeeze them, many mice and rats run inside the compressor. So the compressor squeezes not just the oranges but everything and anything in there as well. Now I will never drink any commercial juice again either.

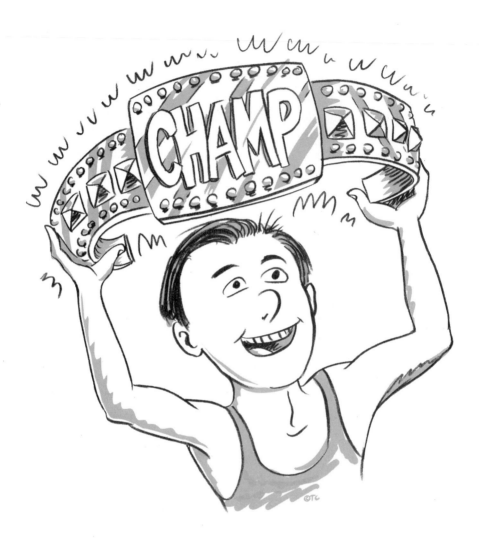

When you beat Cooked Food Man you will be the Champion of Health!

The Raw Foods Glossary

Natural Food: Any food in its natural form. Examples are fruits, vegetables, nuts and seeds. It is best to eat these foods as fresh and as close to the time they were picked as possible. Fresh foods are loaded with health-maintaining vitamins minerals and enzymes—the best foods for the human body.

Sprouted Food: Seeds, nuts, grains, peas and beans sprout when soaked in water, making them easier to digest.

Fermented Food: Foods that have been cultured and fermented to produce friendly bacteria, which will aid the body in knocking out unhealthy bacteria. Examples are miso, seed cheeses and a fermented drink called rejuvelac.

Dehydrated Food: When you dry foods, you take the water content out of the food. If dried at temperatures less than 110 degrees, the enzymes are not destroyed and the food is still considered live or raw. Many people use dehydrated foods to replace the taste of cooked foods in their diet. Examples of dehydrated foods are raw sprouted bread, crackers, candies and dried fruits.

Sea Vegetables: Examples are dulse, nori and kelp. Some raw fooders don't consider Sea Vegetables food for human consumption, while others consider them a very important part of a raw diet as they are rich in minerals and trace elements.

Wild Foods: This includes foods that are found in the wild. representing nature in its purest form—the most nutritious foods people can eat. They include wild vegetables, fruits, nuts, seeds, berries and herbs. There are hundreds of fascinating wild foods in parks, forests, backyards and many other places which people overlook everyday..

Fruits to Know

We all know about great tasting fruits we see everyday: pineapples, avocados, oranges and bananas. These fruits are good, but there are so many more exotic fruits that most people have never heard of. In fact, there is such a variety of different fruits in the world that you could eat a different fruit everyday for the rest of your life and still not even come close to tasting all of them. Let us learn about some of these great tasting fruits.

Durian: If I had to describe it, I would say that it looks like an oversized deformed pineapple. Actually, it has a green to brown shell with spiky pines sticking out of it. On the inside, it has a sweet yellow flesh and big pits. Durian is sweet and juicy with custard-like consistency. It is known for its strong smell. Many people say it tastes like heaven but smells like hell. Durian is grown in Thailand and Malaysia and is shipped frozen to Asian Markets around the world. The durian is one of the most expensive fruits you will ever see, but it tastes so good that it is well worth it. Durian is known as the "king of fruits"

Water coconut: Big green coconut with jelly inside that you can eat with a spoon. They are the same coconuts you see in the stores with brown hair on them, before they get that way. The water inside the coconut is also referred to as coconut water. It is one of the most nutritious liquid on the earth. It is the one food that a person can live on exclusively if in the right environment. It is also called a baby coconut or a young coconut. It is sold in Latin stores or in Asian markets. They grow on just about every tropical island.

Mangosteen: The small purple brown mangosteen cracks open to reveal tasty white segments with a very fine flavor. Mangosteen are known as the "queen of the fruits." They are grown in Southeast Asia.

Jackfruit: An enormous yellow-green fruit that can weigh over 50 lbs. Inside are hundreds of individual bright yellow or orange segments. The texture is slightly rubbery and it tastes like tutti -fruity bubble gum. Jackfruit grows in Florida, Hawaii, the Caribbean and Southeast Asia.

Starfruit: This star-shaped fruit tastes cool, crisp and watery. It comes from Asia but also grows in Florida.

Mamey: On the outside, a mamey looks like a big potato, on the inside it has orange flesh like an avocado surrounded by a big pit. It is very sweet and filling amd tastes like a combination of pumpkin, cherries and strawberries.

Sapodilla: Looks like a small potato. On the inside, it is brown with the texture of a non-crispy, juicy pear. It tastes like a mixture of caramel and honey. Sapodilla grows in the Caribbean where it is called naseberry as well as in Asia, where it is known as Che Che.

Cherimoya: Also known as a custard apple, cherimoya has a thick creamy taste and is green on the outside. Some varieties have many bumps, and some have finger like imprints. It grows in tropical and sub-tropical climates.

White Sapote: On the outside, this fruit is round and yellow. On the inside, it is white and has the consistency of a soft apple. It tastes like vanilla pudding and grows in tropical and sub-tropical climates.

Black Sapote: Brown and soft when ripe, it. is also known as the "chocolate pudding fruit" because it looks and tastes like chocolate pudding. It grows in tropical climates.

ORGANIC FOODS

Organic food should be the only food you put into your body. Organic foods are foods that are not treated with deadly sprays and chemicals. Also, the soil in which organic food is grown has not been sprayed for at least seven years. No matter how good a diet you eat, if the food you are putting into your body is not organic, it will contain harmful chemicals, sprays and waxes that will be detrimental to your health. Organic foods taste much better than eating chemicals. Nature always tastes better than the chemical medicine taste of inorganic foods. These chemicals are not only bad for our health, but they also destroy the environment. What that means is that organic foods will help preserve nature. For you to be the true champion that you are, and stay there, it would be a wise decision to eat organic foods whenever possible. If you have to eat non-organic foods, here are two helpful lists. The first list I suggest you *never* eat from when they're non-organic; the second list is OK to eat if you choose to if organic varieties are not readily available.

**Never eat unless organic
The most heavily sprayed foods are:**

Raisins

Peanuts

Strawberries

Apples

Cantaloupe

Broccoli

Grapes

Leafy Green Vegetables

Cucumbers

Peaches

**OK to eat if non-organic
The least sprayed foods are:**

Coconuts

Avocados

Papayas

Pineapples (US only)

Watermelon

Durians (Malaysian only)

Mangos

Nuts

"People ask me: how can you eat only raw foods in the winter? Aren't you cold? My response is: how can you eat cooked foods in the summer? Aren't you hot?"

—Enrique Candioti

THE RAW DIET, TRY IT!

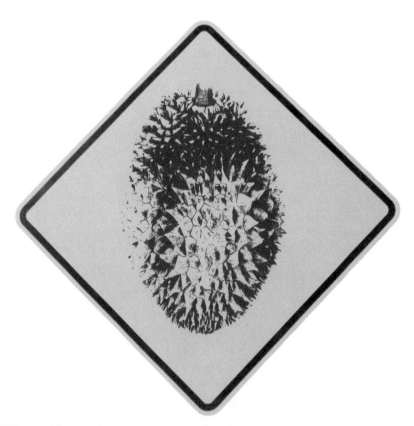

Warning! This is what a durian fruit looks like. Smells like heaven and tastes like heaven! If you see this call the author Paul Nison immediately!

5 | RAW GOAL

My Raw Life

This chapter describes my eating patterns and my health lifestyle. I have been experimenting with and studying the raw-food lifestyle for many years and have put together these guidelines to help myself thrive. I would call these ideas a realistic goal for anyone wanting to advance from the average raw lifestyle to the next level. It is my personal guideline. As you can see, it is much stricter than what previous chapters in this book have suggested. After you have defeated Cooked Food Man, and some time has passed, you may want to make your own chart like this.

When taking your diet to the next level, make it a personal change. There is no need to tell anyone what you are doing, just do it! It is OK to make adjustments along the way. If you want to thrive in life, don't settle for the average, keep moving ahead. This is what will separate you from everyone else.

My Diet

Organic Fruits; Whole. I believe whole fruits are the best for me and also for people in general. Whole fruit is fruit in its purest form, and is the best possible food for man. I don't limit myself to just certain fruits. Anything that has a seed is a fruit. Pepper, tomato, cucumber, and squash are all considered fruits. Whole fruit is always best. Sometimes I like to have a fruit juice too, but not too often. If I do have fruit in juice form, I will dilute it with water so it's not too sweet for me.

Leafy Greens: Whole or juiced. I love to eat leafy green vegetables. Kale is my favorite. Many people ask me how I can just eat it plain with no dressing. When I first became raw, I didn't like it, but the taste grew on me. Now I love it. I know some raw fooders who don't eat any leafy greens. If they feel that is best, then fine. I think greens are important, but it is more important to eat what you like and not to eat what doesn't taste good to you.

Whole **Sea vegetables** It took a lot for me to get used to them. First I had to get used to the idea of eating them, then to the taste. I meet raw fooders who say it's not natural to eat sea vegetables. Once again, if you don't like the taste, don't eat them. Now I've come to liking the taste, and I have spoken with many long-time raw fooders who also believe sea vegetables are very important to have in the diet.

Other vegetables: Eat sparingly. Leafy greens are the only vegetables I eat on a daily basis. They contain the energy of the sun which is then passed along to me when I eat them. All other vegetables are not as easy to digest. I do like to eat them, but sparingly.

Nuts and Seeds. I always try to soak nuts and seeds before I eat them. I feel they are much better for my body that way. I rarely used to soak them, but since I began soaking them, I now see a big difference. When soaked, nuts and seeds digest much easier and faster. Also, whenever I eat them, I try to buy them in the shell. This helps me to avoid overeating on nuts. I try not to eat more than three handfuls a week. Sometimes I will go months without any. If I crave more, I blend and strain them to make nut milk. I love the taste of nut milk. It is also very filling. Many people tend to overeat on nuts, so be careful not to eat too many nuts.

Dried Fruit. It is best to eat food that contains as much water as possible. Except for dates, I only eat dried fruits if I can't get them fresh. Eating fruits in their most natural state is always best. I also like to soak dried fruit, to replace the water, before I eat them. I try never to eat more than three handfuls in a week. I can go for months without them.

The best diet for me is to eat as little as possible. The more I get into eating frugally, the easier it becomes to do this. Right now I eat, on the average, two meals per day or less. When I eat two meals, my first meal is usually fresh juicy fruits. The second meal consists of leafy greens and fatty fruits such as avocadoes. I always do my best to combine my foods well. Most of the time, I eat a mono diet so I don't have to worry about improper food combining. I also avoid eating too much fatty fruits. I often go a few days without eating any.

Eating

Avoid overeating. I think that overeating is the biggest problem that people have, especially people who are new to the raw food lifestyle. It is a big problem with cooked food eaters as well. I think everyone overeats. I do all I can to avoid it.

Eat only one kind of fat per day. I think the hardest

food to digest is fatty food. I feel the body does much better when it only has to deal with one kind of fat at a time. For example, if I eat an avocado, that would be my fatty food for the day. I will eat no other fats, no nuts, olives, etc. on that day. This works best for me.

I advise everyone to experiment and learn. No two people are in the same situation. What works for me might not work for you. But raw food can work for everyone, no matter where they are. I don't know anyone else who eats only one kind of fat per day, and I have never heard anyone talk about it, but I feel that for my body, it is best. I feel my digestion works best when I eat it this way. I call this way of eating, "Mono Fat." As it takes a longer time for my body to digest fats than other nutrients, I try not to eat fatty foods everyday. I feel eating fatty foods no more than 3 or 4 times a week is fine for me. When I started on a raw diet, I ate fatty foods more frequently.

Eat only during daylight. By eating only during daylight hours and almost never eating at night, I keep myself from over-eating and from engaging in late-night binges. This took a lot of getting used to, but now that I am used to it, this health practice is very beneficial. I have never felt better in my life, and I owe a big part of the improvement to this practice. Of course, if I feel true hunger, I will eat, regardless of the time.

Don't eat two fruit meals in a row. For a while, I was overeating on sweet fruits and couldn't stop. Every meal was sweet fruit, sweet fruit, sweet fruit. Then Dr. Fred Bisci taught me how eating too much fruit increases blood gases (see his interview). He suggested avoiding eating two fruit meals in a row. Like every thing that makes sense to me, I tried it and it worked. I now eat more greens in my diet.

Drink a great deal of water upon arising, and throughout the day. I learned about this practice from Morris Krok. I always try to get the cleanest water available. I use distilled water from glass bottles. There are so many benefits of doing this that I could write a whole additional book on the benefits. For one, drinking lots of water helps clean and flush out the body. Another great benefit is it gives me such a feeling of fullness that I don't feel like eating until the middle of the day. I think everyone should try drinking a lot of water upon arising for one week. When you wake up, drink 6 to 10 glasses of water at room temperature, plus lots of additional water throughout the day. If you do this, food will be the last thing on your mind, and you will have a difficult time overeating. Morris is a genius.

Think before you eat. Before eating a particular food, first ask yourself these questions: Am I hungry? Do I really want to eat this? In the wild, would I be able to eat this food without utensils? If you answered no to any of these, don't eat it. I think it is best to eat something only after asking these questions. If the answer yes to all these questions, I enjoy my meals even more.

Concentrate on the food. I make a big effort to put all of my attention on the food I am about to eat.

Avoid talking when you have food in your mouth. I think it is important to fully focus the mind on the act of eating food. food. I find I can't properly concentrate and chew food correctly if I am talking. I don't think anyone can. I enjoy my food much more when I don't talk while eating.

Follow food combining guidelines. For best digestion I follow the food combing guidelines if I am not eating a meal of just one kind of food (A mono meal) .

Have a fun meal. Every now and then, I allow myself to eat a meal where foods may happen to be improperly combined. I don't do this often, but it's good to know that if I want to have fun once in a while with my food, I can. Too much strictness can be dangerous. If I have too much fun, I know I will feel it the next day. Therefore, I try not to go overboard. I always think ahead.

Cleansing

Fruits with seeds are more cleansing than fruits with pits. Seed-fruits such as grapes go through my body much better than pit-fruits such as peaches. I believe they are more cleansing. I know many people who feel the same way.

Skin brush your body. I try to skin brush often. Everyday is best as the skin is a major organ of elimination. I recommend going to a health food store and buying a skin brush. A skin brush looks like a brush you would use in the shower, but instead, you brush your skin when it is dry.

Fasting. I fast whenever I feel I need too. I have learned to read my body, so even if I feel fine, I can tell when some part of my body needs to rest. I always fast when I feel rundown. I monitor this through my sleeping patterns, bowel movements and other bodily signs.

"No one knows your body better than you do."

Speaking

Only speak positive words. I always try my best to think before I speak. And when I do speak, I only speak positively: This is much harder to do than it sounds yet it is a lot of fun, like learning a new language.

Sleeping & Rest

When I wake up, if I feel like going back to sleep, then I know I didn't have enough sleep. When I wake up, I should want to jump out of bed and start the day. If I don't want to, it is a sure sign I did not get enough good sleep.

If I feel tired, I try to take a rest or a nap during the day. I need to have the time to do this; it helps so much. I think a big problem with society is that, because of rigid work schedules, people can't sleep and rest when their bodies need it. People are forced to sleep by the clock and not by the body's inner wisdom. This leads to stress and toxemia.

Don't use an alarm clock. This is bad habit. I try my best to not to wake up to an alarm clock. Shocking the system too abruptly in order to wake up destroys some of the benefits of good sleep. Waking up by an alarm clock is the equivalent of going on a water diet (water fast) and breaking it with pizza! Waking to an alarm is harmful and unnatural to the human body, but because of the demands of society (i.e.not being late for work) many people use alarm clocks.

Exercising

Engage in some form of exercise everyday, if you have the time. If I received enough sleep the night before, I love to do calisthenics and yoga every morning,

If you feel tired when waking up, you did not get enough sleep. If I am tired in the morning and don't feel like getting up, I stay in bed. I don't push myself. I will use that extra time to sleep and skip exercising that day.

"When you are in attune with ideas emanating from within you, you will be ahead, always ahead."

—Morris Krok

6 | RAW SURVIVAL

The New Contenders

You are a champion now. You are on top of the world and it feels too good to want to go back to being a shell of a champion. Like all champions, however, you will have to defend your title. Many newcomers will try to take your title from you. Cooked Food Man is still very upset that you beat him. He will do anything for a rematch. No matter what happens from here on out, do not give him or any of your other opponents another chance to hurt you again. They all have been trying to hurt you. Some of them have even tried to kill you. But you survived. Cooked Food Man is poison. Leave him and the rest of his friends where they belong—in the past. Don't make them part of your future.

Move on and face the newcomers who will try to take your title away from you. Learning Man, Language Man, Willpower Man, Change Man, Mind Man and the rest of your support crew have been a big help up to now. They will always be there for you and they will all be needed to defeat the new challengers that wait for you.

The challenges you will have to meet are different now because you are the champion. Before you had your life to lose and your health to gain. Now you have your newfound health to lose. Everyone will try to take your title from you. To defeat these opponents, you will have to add an extra trainer to your corner crew, a specialist, to help you deal with these new contenders. His name is Detoxification Man. He was hired to help you defeat them. Make sure you listen to him and understand everything he teaches you. If you can understand his message and trust him, you will never have any problems from any of your contenders ever again. If you ignore Detoxification Man's important training, you will lose your title.

It's now time to meet Detoxification Man as well as meet the new contenders who will try to take away the title that you worked so hard to get. You are no longer a challenger, you are a champion. Go get them!

Detoxification Man

Detoxification Man will train you like no other trainer can because he is a specialist. Most trainers just guide you. Detoxification Man will get in the ring himself and spar with you. He is just as strong as your other sparring partner, Mind Man. Mind Man is the only one who ever beat Detoxification Man in a real battle. They are friends now and, although things sometimes get a little rough between them, they will always be friends. They both only want to help you and see you get and stay well. Once you are hit by a few of Detoxification Man's understanding punches, you will realize this. If you can't beat him you will never beat your new contenders.

To beat Detoxification Man, you have to understand and accept the natural process of detoxification. Otherwise, he will beat you by forcing you to give up. Show him love. Accept that he is not your enemy but your friend, no matter how he might appear. Realize that he is not trying to hurt you, that although he keeps hitting you, he is really helping you. All he needs is some TLC and understanding. He was only hired to help you beat your new opponents. Let him teach you what he has to, to clean you out, and then he will go away and leave you to soak in his benefits.

Detoxification Man is so ugly that people will try to make you think he only wants to hurt you. Those people are from Cooked Food Man's support crew, so don't listen to them. Cooked Food Man sent them to try to fool you, but you are too smart for that. Let's hear what Learning Man has to teach us about Detoxification Man.

Learning Man says, *"you have to know all about the changes that your body will go through when you become Raw Food Man or Raw Food Woman."* When you become a champion, many positive changes will happen to your body, *but you will feel worse before you feel better, and you will look worse before you look better*. This process is known as a detoxification or a healing crisis. Some people's detoxification crises are more severe than others. The more toxic you were before you became a champion, the worse the symptoms will be. If you don't understand what is happening, and don't accept the changes, you will not be able to handle the punches from Detoxification Man and you will give up. You will only be able to deal with these changes by understanding them.

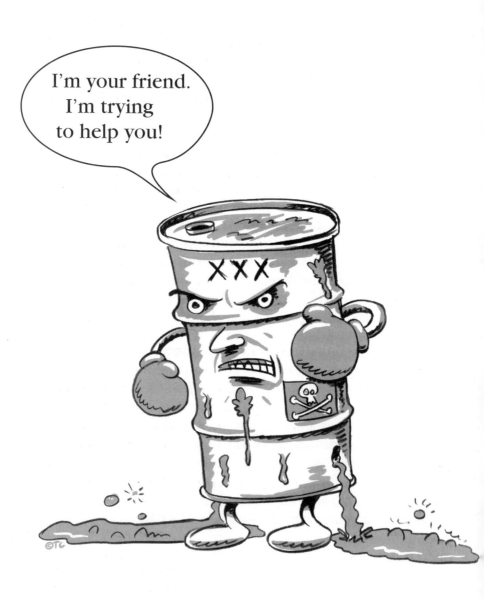

Detoxification Man

Let us list some of the changes that your body may go through: Past opponents may reappear and give you one last punch. Legal Drug Man may show up again and try to get another fight with you. You must not give him a chance to fight you again. It would be wise to just ignore the fact that he is even there. When you get signs of a healing crisis (which often happens when you first become a champion), don't take any aspirins or other over the counter drugs. Definitely do not take any medication from a doctor—antibiotics especially, as they are the worst. (They work against, not with, the body).

The changes that your body goes through during a healing crisis are good. They show that your body is working to get rid of all the bad toxins that do not belong inside of you. The changes might not feel good, but don't worry. Once you have defeated your new opponents and become clean, Detoxification Man will leave, and you will feel terrific.

When your body is detoxifying, it is getting rid of all the waste that you had put inside before you became a champion. Detoxification symptoms will be different for each person. Your body will use whatever ways it can find to get rid of unnatural toxins. For some people it might be a headache, for others, it might be a cold or a skin rash. It might be more serious; it could even be cancer or other life-threatening diseases (toxemia). *While you are eating a raw diet, all changes will be positive, no matter how bad they might seem*. When your body is in the process of getting rid of toxins, it is cleaning itself.

A big problem people often have with a healing crisis is that once they experience any sign of discomfort, they begin to think that what they were doing was wrong. They let Detoxification Man beat them at that point. Instead of going with the flow and understanding what is happening, people just give up and go back to their old habits that brought them to the point of discomfort in the first place. They go back to being unnatural. To survive the ongoing stages of detoxification over time, become friends with Detoxification Man and welcome these changes.

The fastest and quickest way would be to go on a water-only diet (water fast). But this would also be the most painful and intense way, because toxins might be released too fast into your system. It might be too extreme for very toxic people.

There are ways to make the symptoms of detoxification less painful and less stressful to your body. One option to slow the symptoms and pains of a detoxification is to go on a liquid diet or eat very lightly. Some light, juicy citrus fruits or melons will slow the symptoms down a little. However, the symptoms will last a little longer. If that is still too hard on your body, you could add other light fruits like papaya or apple.

Learning Man says that when you go through a detoxification, you are going to look worse before you look better. You might lose weight and look thin to others and yourself. You might get pimples, or your skin might turn pale. You might even begin to smell badly as the toxins start coming out. This is all part of the detoxification process. If you "go with the flow," and get through the healing crisis, afterwards your skin will actually start to develop a glow. You will put on the weight you lost, your complexion will become an amazingly beautiful color, and your body will smell clean and fresh. Each round you successfully train with Detoxification Man, you get stronger in all ways.

Now is the time to reject panic and ride it out. It is also the time to make sure Willpower Man is close by your side. Stay focused and seek out people who have been there, and who understand. They will be your Support Crew and they will help get you through this period. You worked hard to get here. Don't let anyone tell you how you should live. You are the champion now. It is your title to keep. When you are done training with Detoxification Man, the hardest part will be over. Stay focused and have fun always. Keep studying, keep reading and keep winning.

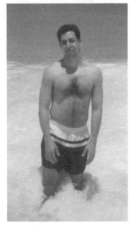

Paul cooked

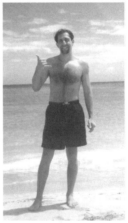

Paul raw

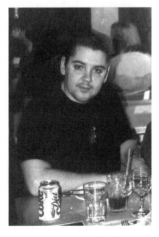

Enrique cooked

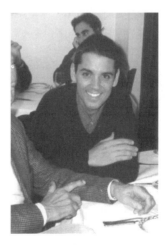

Enrique raw

Skin brushing

Skin brushing aids the body in cleansing. It removes dead skin from your body and assists the body in getting rid of toxins. It also helps the movement of lymph flow in the body. I highly recommend you take five minutes a day to skin brush for best health. I promise you more than just your skin will benefit.

Underweight Man

Also known as Weight Losing Man, this contender used to be in the corner of Detoxification Man, but he became so powerful and beat so many people that he went out on his own. He is the next contender who will try to destroy you and take away your title. Don't let him get to you. He will try to get as many people as he can to line up against you. To knock him out, you will have to hit him with your understanding punch. If you learn about the human body and the effects of detoxification, cleansing and healing upon it, you will understand why you are losing weight. Once you do, nothing that anyone says or does will make you want to give up your title.

Learning Man tells you, that when it comes to beating Weight Losing Man, your best offense is your defense. As long as you do not let Weight Losing Man hit you, you are going to win. Weight Losing Man will try many different ways to get to you, but as long as you stay focused and understand what is happening, he won't be able to hurt you. Learn how your body works and why it loses weight when you start eating a raw-food diet. I will give you some information, but the best way to gain this understanding is to read and study what is already available to you. Many good books demonstrate that losing weight at the beginning of a raw-food diet is a necessary part of the healing process. Weight Losing Man is just another contender, and when you beat him, you will be a much stronger champion than you are today.

Before you even convince yourself that you are underweight, consider the possibility that before you went on the raw-food diet you were overweight, and that now your weight is fine. The reason most people think they are too skinny is not because of how they themselves feel about their own looks, but because of what other people tell them. If you were alone, you would most likely think you always look fine or you wouldn't give any thought to how you look. Your mind and your body are one unit that works together as a whole. It breaks down and it heals as one unit.

By now, hopefully you understand that cooked food is poison. The cooked food you have eaten all this time has clogged your body and caused toxins to build up inside. Once your body has cleansed, healed and is ready, it will put back any weight it needs. You have to be patient and strong-minded. You might not put back as much weight as you lost, but if you were on the SAD (Standard American Diet) you probably were overweight

Underweight Man

159

anyway. If you were underweight, once your body cleans out, you will put on the weight that you were never able to gain before as you will be better able to assimilate your food.

Stay strong and focused. Your body will do the rest. It is an amazing machine, and it knows what it is doing. You just have to let it function properly. Assist your body, but try not to interfere with its work.

Don't complain about weight-loss, or try to put on weight by eating often or by consuming fatty foods. This makes no sense and will actually keep you from putting on weight. It doesn't matter how much you eat, if the body is not clean, it cannot efficiently assimilate the food. Overeating will clog your body even more. If you give your body more to clean, it will have to work harder and take longer to return to normal.

"We gain benefit from our food, not in proportion to the amount we eat, but in the amount we can properly utilize and assimilate."

— Dr. Hereward Carrington from *Fasting for Health and Long Life*

Don't worry about how you look. As I said about detoxification, you will look worse before you look better. When the time comes, you will reach the point where your body will wake up and be ready to start putting on weight. Have patience and wait for that time. If you can do that, then you have just knocked out Underweight Man. Congratulations! Go to your next opponent.

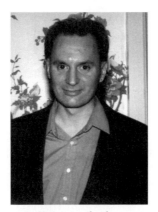

Gary cooked.

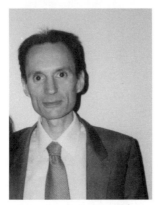

Gary at begining of detox.
Massive weight loss.

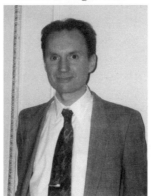

Gary raw. After detox,
weight comes back.

Overeating Man

It's true—too much of even a *good* thing is bad. Even with natural foods, you can overeat. Because natural foods taste so delicious, it is very easy to eat them to excess. If you overeat, the extra food will burden your system. It won't be as harmful as overeating on unnatural processed and cooked foods, but it will hurt you and will make you lose your title to Overeating Man.

Overeating Man is a tricky opponent. He will try to keep you happy while he beats you up. His big knockout punch is his taste punch. He knows all the opponents you have beaten in the past and what a great champion you have become. He knows that you are eating many great tasting fruits, vegetables and nuts. He will try to take advantage of that. He will try to trick you into thinking he is your friend. If you let him, he will beat you. The more you overeat, the more you jeopardize losing your title as champion of the world. And you will also lose your new name, Raw Food Man or Raw Food Woman.

As I said earlier, the best way to eat and make sure that Overeating Man never defeats you is to consume a mono diet. This means to eat one food at a time. If you mix your food, everything you eat will taste good to you all the time, making it very easy to overeat.

"When you feed your body what it needs, your internal fluids stay in balance, your cells are fed and your body is healthy. Disease, on the other hand, happens when your body is overtaxed, attempting to clean non-nutritious food out of your system. Then your cells starve and eventually die and so do you. Food that does not directly benefit the body is treated as waste."

—Roe Gallo, *Perfect Body*

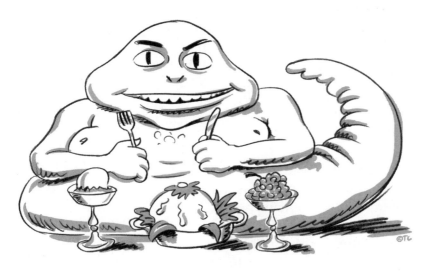

Overeating Man

To beat Overeating Man, plan out your diet. Have all the food that you are going to eat in one day either on the table or in your mind. As long as you plan your meals wisely, it is hard to overeat.

Another way you will beat Overeating Man is by abstaining from food at night for at least 12 to 14 hours. Eat only during the daylight hours. This way, even if you do tend to overeat, your body will have enough time to recuperate and break down all that food and, most importantly, to rest. So make sure you do your best to only eat during daylight hours.

"If food is eaten before the last meal has been digested, trouble is bound to follow."

—Dr. Hereward Carrington from his book *Fasting For Health and Long Life*

In modern society, most people overeat, yet don't realize how much they do. On the average, when a person goes on an extended water fast, he will lose one pound of body weight per day. This would mean that, to maintain his natural weight, he would have to eat only one pound of food a day, yet people eat much more than that. These numbers are not precise, but very close, and give a good illustration of the extent to which many people overeat.

When we consider the amount of extra food we eat that the body doesn't need, plus the poor quality of the food, it is no wonder why so many people become toxic. If all this food causes disease (toxemia), it is obvious that the cure would be to stop eating so much. This is so simple, yet so hard for many people to understand, not to mention accomplish. "Overeating even the highest quality raw foods will still cause toxemia in the body."

Overeating is not natural to the human body. The body needs very little food, much less than people realize. Overeating is a bad habit people learn in their early childhood. Parents force-feed their babies so they eat more, and the resulting habit stays with us all our life unless we break it.

Just as a baby spits out food when he is overfed, the body will also release the food it can't use. This is what disease (toxemia) actually is. It is the body trying to get rid of food for which it has no use. This extra food is waste. When a person stops overeating, the body is given time to get rid of this waste and revert to a healthy state. When people continue to overeat, as some people do on a daily basis, the body can never achieve a state of health. It will continue to build more waste till the body loses its power to push it out. That is the final stage of toxemia. I am convinced that if we took all the people, in all of the hospitals, educated them and put them on a supervised fast, 99% of them would heal and remain in the best of health. Of course, if we did this, the doctors and drug companies would fail to make any money, so I don't really expect it to happen. This is why we must educate ourselves and take our health into our own hands.

Once you understand overeating is a bad habit that you must control in order to be in the best of health, you have taken a huge step in the right direction. Anytime you abuse a habit you form an addiction. Both the habit and the addiction can and must be broken to avoid toxemia. The best way to break a bad habit is with a good habit. Replace the overeating habit with positive thoughts and with new healthy habits. Spend extra time with Willpower Man if you must. Also, spend time with Change Man. They will help you break those habits.

There are many reasons people overeat. Often, they are eating just out of habit and not on the basis of their true nutritional needs. If they were, they would eat only a few times a week at most. Thought and mood can be a cause. Eating while experiencing certain feelings can cause you to overeat and lose to Overeating Man.

Timing is also a big factor. A common reason people overeat is that they eat at the wrong time. If you want to beat Overeating Man, never eat when you are angry, anxious, fearful or upset. Eating during these times leaves you wide open to getting knocked out by Overeating Man.

In addition, many people tend to overeat because of boredom. Stay busy at all times. Spend your time wisely and you will win. If you get careless and let boredom slip into your life, you will set yourself up for disaster.

Many people overeat when they are depressed. Again, if you ever feel depressed for any reason, seek out your corner crew. They, and not food, will help you beat Overeating Man. Avoid the depression punch. If you let it hit you, it will knock you out and take your title away. Overeating Man will hit you with punches every now and then but they will not hurt you. You are a tough champion. As long as you understand and stay focused, you will beat Overeating Man and stay the champion. Knock him out and go on to your next opponent.

> The best time to eat is when true hunger exists. That is only right after an extended water fast when your appetite comes back. If you are not able to do a long fast, the best time to eat would be when you feel you need food, not when you want food. There is a difference between needing and wanting. Learn the difference and you will never overeat.

Frozen Food Man

Another newcomer you will have to watch out for, who will try to beat you, is Frozen Food Man. Many people will try to make you believe that frozen foods are good for you and that they are not processed in anyway. The truth is that frozen foods are less harmful than cooked or heat-destroyed foods, but they are still processed and unnatural to eat. When a food is frozen at a certain temperature, its enzymes start to deteriorate, thus destroying the quality of the food.

Judging by taste and food composition, there are some frozen foods that hold up better than other frozen foods. When you start eating naturally, you might crave certain frozen foods. Eating them sparingly would be okay. However, if you want to lose the taste for them completely, you will have to completely stop consuming them. You are a champion and you will, in time, eliminate your intake of all frozen foods, thus defeating Frozen Food Man. Then you will never look back.

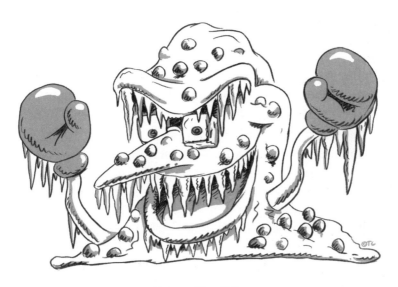

Frozen Food Man

Many Exotic Fruits are Frozen Food?

Many exotic fruits from other countries, especially South East Asia, are frozen before they are shipped to the United States. There are a few reasons for this. First, the fruits ripen very quickly. If they arrived in their fresh form, they would spoil too quickly. Second, and most importantly, the U.S. government prohibits certain fresh fruits from entering the country because of the danger of invading bugs that would have "hitchhiked" on the fruit. There are so many great fresh fruits from around the world that most of us have never tasted. However, although these great fresh fruits can't come to you, if possible, try to *go to them* by traveling to where they grow. Examples of exotic fruits which are frozen are durians, mangosteens, lyches, etc. These fruits are usually found in Asian or Hispanic markets, and not in regular local grocery stores.

You will meet many newcomer challengers in the future. I just named a few of the more obvious ones. Your corner crew, and everything that you have learned, will help you. If things ever get too out of hand, Willpower Man will always be there, as long as you use him. If you choose to avoid him, he will go away. Make good use of him and keep educating yourself. Keep track of all the opponents that you beat for future reference. More importantly, keep information on any opponents that beat you, so you will know what to look out for if you ever have to fight them again.

Once again, congratulations! You are the champion; nobody can beat you but yourself. Move on to the next chapter and always be ready for one of the old opponents that you have already defeated. They will try to fight you again. Don't give your attention to any of them and they will go away. As long as you always remain ready for them, you can never be surprised.

> Natural is simplicity in its purest form.

7 | RAW NATURE BEING AS NATURAL AS YOU CAN BE

The unnatural exposed!

You have now beaten all the newcomers that deal directly with food. There will now be some new challenges you must face to keep growing as a champion. You have already switched to natural foods; now you should strive to move as close to nature as possible in other aspects of your life. Understanding what is happening in the world will automatically get you even closer to nature.

To understand what being natural really is, imagine being stranded on an island. Imagine you were born on this island. I am not talking about a small island with one tree, like you see in cartoons. I am talking about a big island, the size of one of the Hawaiian islands. Think about how you would have to live if you lived according to the laws of nature. Things that you wouldn't have on that island are things that you don't need to survive today. You know that you will need clothes, because in society, you are not permitted to go without them. But you do have a choice of what clothes you choose to wear. Choose fibers that are as natural as possible and wear as little as possible and still be comfortable. If you live in a warm climate, this

169

will be easy. It can also be done in a cold climate; adjust this plan to your needs. Just wear as little as possible to stay warm and comfortable, and always wear loose fitting clothes to allow your skin to breath.

Many things in your life are unnatural. Let's look at some of the more obvious ones you rely upon. You probably don't realize how unnatural they really are.

"The more you eat raw food, the less material things you need for survival in life."

Television. One way to describe a television is that it is a brainwashing machine. If you were on that previously mentioned paradise island, you would enjoy all the great beauty nature has to offer. Think of what you would miss if you had a television. If they had TV on Gilligan's island, who would have built the huts and everything else they made? Nobody, because they all would have been watching television. Nothing would have gotten done.

This is what television does to people. It programs them to become lazy. Why do you think they call it programming? Many people waste their lives in front of the television/brainwashing machine.

You shouldn't watch entertainment; you should *be* entertainment. Go outside and do something, anything. Just stay away from that unnatural brainwasher. People always say they do not have enough time in the day to get everything done, but then they watch many hours of television. Ninety percent of the junk you see on television consists of negative messages anyway, and you watch them without even realizing it. Television is a poison, an addictive, unnatural brainwashing toxin that you do not need in your new natural, pleasant, simple lifestyle. One day you will realize this for yourself, if you haven't already. That day you will beat Television Man and when you do, you will not just be a champion, but you will also be a legend.

Makeup and Beauty Lotions. Women are literally "dying" to look beautiful these days. When will they realize that the only true beauty is natural beauty? Anyone who wears any kind of makeup at all is putting deadly toxins into the largest elimination system of the body, the skin. They are also stopping toxins from exiting. This applies not just to makeup alone but to all beauty supplies. When you become a champion, you will realize that you do not need to put deadly chemicals into your body to look beautiful. Once you eat 100% raw foods and stop polluting your body with unnatural substances such as makeup, you will have the nicest skin that anyone has ever seen. If you beat all the opponents, but are still wearing makeup and lotions, you will lose your title.

You do not want to lose your championship title to Makeup Woman. She will beat you just as badly as all the other opponents. She has a secret punch. She makes everyone think that there is nothing wrong with wearing makeup, and that it is an absolute must if you want to look good. After years and years of taking her punches, her punches will catch up to you. If you let her keep beating you, she will hurt you and take your title away.

If you want to be natural, you have to be completely natural. There is nothing natural about Makeup Woman. If you still don't think that all make-up is bad for you, take a stick of lipstick or mascara and eat it. You would not even think of actually doing this because you know that all these chemicals would make you sick if you put them inside of your body. Well, where do you think they are going when you put them on your skin? They are still going into your body, and they are making you sick. If you want to be a beautiful, loving person, always remember that to love other people, you have to first love yourself. There is no need to cover your beautiful face with makeup. Makeup is for clowns in the circus, not for beautiful people like you. Stop putting that mask on your face everyday and be the beautiful, natural champion that you were meant to be!

> Let us make a natural rule:
> If you can't eat it, don't use it on your body.

Sunglasses. You have been misled into thinking that sunglasses will protect your eyes from the sun. Sunglasses actually make you more susceptible to sunburn and skin cancer. Roe Gallo explains this best in *Perfect Body*. "*Sunglasses are particularly bad for you. The body is partially protected from the rays of the sun because of your body's natural perception of the sun's brightness. When it is let in through a smaller opening. In the back of the pupil are melanin cells. When the sun's rays contact the release dark pigment throughout the entire body to protect the skin from sun damage. When you wear sunglasses, the darkness of the glass fools your eyes, interfering with your natural skin protection. Burning and skin cancer are the result.*" If you want to be as natural as you can be and remain a champion, only wear sunglasses when you must—in dangerous glare situations, such as in snow skiing or when driving your car while facing the glaring sun.

> If you want to become truly natural, you have to be 100% natural in everything you do. Everyone can achieve it. If you think you cannot, you just don't want to.

Toothpaste. If you ever read the writing on a common commercial toothpaste tube, it says "do not let children ingest." It also says to put only a pea-sized amount of toothpaste on the toothbrush. Toothpaste is not only unnatural, it is also a waste of your hard-earned money. It consists primarily of flavoring to disguise the odor of your breath; it is not really for your teeth at all. When you become clean on the inside, you will never have bad breath to worry about and you will not need toothpaste anymore. When you eat 100% natural food, as long as you brush and floss and limit citrus and dried fruits, your teeth will be fine. Be natural and be clean. Brush your teeth without using toothpaste. Also, floss your teeth everyday. Even flossing and the use of a brush are not truly natural, but because of the way our jaws are constructed, we must aid them in some way to keep them healthy.

> Don't be fooled by the word natural. Nothing you see on a store shelf, in a box, bottle or a tube is in a natural form. Only products found in nature are natural.

Perfumes, colognes, mouthwash and deodorant. Everyone wants to smell good. Some people are "dying" to do so. Everyday millions of people are putting poisons into their bodies when they use these products. These deadly poisons are just toxic chemicals with a pretty name.

When you become all natural, there will be no need to cover up your body's odor or your body's breath. When you try to cover your true body odor, all you are doing is clogging your skin. In this way, you hold in your body the toxins that your body is trying to eliminate through your skin and put more toxins inside your body at the same time. Understand that cooked food, processed food and all the unnatural substances that you put in your body cause foul odors. Without them, you will just have a fresh, natural odor. Think about it. If you eat a dead animal, how do you think it smells inside your body? How will the odor of that dead animal get out of you? It will be through your skin and your breath.

Eat a 100% raw-food diet and you will smell fresh, without the use of these unnatural substances. You will be another step closer to nature.

Eyeglasses and contact lenses. The biggest fraud in the world has to be eyeglasses and contact lenses. Do you see any animals in nature with eyeglasses? Animals have amazing eyesight because they eat only raw foods and live a raw life. Eyeglasses make your eyesight better, but your eyes worse. If you want to restore your eyesight, exercise your eye muscles. In *Perfect Body*, Roe Gallo states: *"vision therapy relaxes and strengthens the eye muscles. Corrective glasses and contact lenses are a crutch. They help you see better temporarily but do not correct your vision. Vision therapy does work, even if someone is considered legally blind. Aldous Huxley and Meir Schnieder are perfect examples. These two high-profile men went from being legally blind to being able to see by practicing vision therapy."*

Roe Gallo regained her eyesight as well and talks about it in her book. I meet more and more people who have done this. It takes time and is a lot of work, but the reward of getting back your eyesight far outweighs the work expended.

There are several excellent books on this subject to help you. (See recommended reading list in the back of this book). I recommend you research vision therapy as much as possible. Get some books, learn the exercises and become natural again.

Hospitals. If you are sick and you want to die, go to the most unnatural environment you can find—a hospital. Everything from hospital food to medical equipment is completely unnatural. Unless you are in dire need of an emergency room, stay away from this environment. Going to a hospital for treatment of anything other than an emergency is like putting the final nail into your coffin. Here is an example. A friend who recently had a heart attack went to a hospital and the first meal they gave him after his triple bypass surgery consisted of pork.

Please stay as far away from hospitals as you can. Understand that doctors are not trained to heal the human body; they are trained in drug therapy. ***The best healer of your body is your own body.*** No one knows your body better than you do. Treat it correctly and it will take care of itself.

The only important part of any hospital is the emergency room, or perhaps the use of plastic surgery after an accident. These are the only ways where the extensive training that doctors receive ever pays off. The problem is that once the emergency is over, patients are not given the chance to get better naturally. If a person could either go home or transfer to a real health institute to heal, this would be a great system. Unfortunately, this is not how it works. Emergency room doctors perform a great job at repairing people, but then send them to other parts of the hospital where they get sick again.

If you feel the need to heal your body and want to become as natural as you can be, I recommend any of several healing centers. These centers will teach you how to become natural again. If you have cancer, arthritis, diabetes or any other disease (toxemia) caused by an unnatural lifestyle and feel the need for a hospital, go to one of these natural healing centers instead. More and more of them are opening up all over the world. Here are some great ones in the United States:

Hippocrates Health Institute
1443 Palmdale Court
West Palm Beach, Florida 33411
561-471-8876

Esser's Ranch
P.O. Box 6229
Lake Worth, Florida 33466
561-965-4360

The Ann Wigmore Institute
PO Box 429
Rincon, Puerto Rico 00677
787-868-6307

Optimum Health Institute
6970 Central Ave
Lemon Grove, CA 91945
619-464-3346

Supplements. There is nothing natural about supplements. They are processed and unnatural, and they are cooked. You should get your vitamins and minerals from your food and from the sun. If you take any supplements, Cooked Food Man is still beating you. Re-evaluate your natural diet and make adjustments. Taking unnatural supplements is never a solution for obtaining vitamins that you feel you are lacking. Add whatever is missing in the form of organic raw foods. People who eat a cooked food diet and then require supplements just offer additional proof that cooked foods are incomplete. No one on a good raw food diet ever needed supplements. The Raw Food Diet has everything you need to be a champion.

Mentally Raw (Mind, spirit and thinking—when you're "natural")

When I first started eating mostly raw food, I did it for health reasons. Until that time in my life, I gave very little thought to spirituality, God or religion. I only believed in science. I used to think that once your body stops working and you die, you cease to exist.

The biggest change in my life since becoming natural has been something that I was not even looking for. Before, I thought life was explained by science, and that was that. Now, 100% of me believes there is more. I now believe in an afterlife and in past lives. This shift has been one of the most amazing feelings in the world.

I know many people who have been eating natural foods for a very long time and they all feel the same way. Someone told me that when you become truly natural, this is a normal process. It is as if your mind had spent the whole unnatural life inside a dirty house, with the windows so dirty that it could not see outside very much. That house is your body. It could only see what was brought inside the house. Then one day you clean your body. This house was like a glass house, but you never noticed it because of the dirt. Now that it is clean, the light of the sun shines through and you can see out of the windows everywhere. Those windows are your mind and once it is clean you will see the truth about everything.

When you become a true champion, you will see how clear everything appears, even things that were vague to you before. You will feel like you are on top of the world and nothing can bring you down. Call it whatever you want to; I call it spirituality. It is hard to see it or understand it when you are not there yet. It will find you when the time is right. How many people can truly say that they feel great, physically and mentally, all the time? You can say that only when you have reached this point. You get to really know and appreciate yourself and your life. You begin to understand where you came from and where you are going.

People today put so much thought into their future that they neglect the present. Take care of yourself. Live by the laws of nature now, and nature will take care of you in the future. When you become natural, you truly become one with yourself. ***You want to be whole and natural in mind and body, a whole person.*** When you are, it is the most amazing feeling in the universe. You do not need to learn to become natural; you have to forget how to be unnatural. Spirituality will take care of everything else. When you feel this way, you will no longer be just a champion. You will be a living legend.

"You should never want more than you need."

"The more you have, the more you have to lose.

To be at peace with yourself and to become a true champion, you must learn not to hold any grudges. You should have no hatred or resentment in your heart or in your thoughts.

Natural child birth, home schooling and bringing up your child 100% natural

Today, many natural women are so pleased with their new natural lives that they want the same quality of life for their newborn babies and young children. One of the greatest moments in a person's life is the birth of their child. I've been told by women that the joy they felt after they gave birth naturally, without any drugs, cannot be measured. All babies should be born this way. The most beautiful thing you will ever witness in your life is a child being born 100% natural through natural childbirth. In her book, *Primal Mothering In A Modern World,* author Hygeia Halfmoon describes everything you need to know about natural child birth. She shares her own experience of natural birth in its purest form. Her book will touch your heart and your mind. If you are, or aspire to be, a natural woman, and are going to have a child, I highly recommend that you read this book.

If you already have a child and want your child to be 100% natural, the earlier in life a person changes to a natural way of living, the easier the change will be for them. The best way to beat any addicting habit is not to get addicted in the first place. How great would it be for your child to be 100% natural and not have to fight any of the opponents you had to fight? Your child would be a champion very early in life. They would be in the best of health. Your child would excel at everything they did in life. They will feel like a champion all of the time. Your child would truly be a natural person in an unnatural world. If you are interested in bringing up your child

100% naturally, there are many books that will teach you more about the subject. (For more information, or to order *Primal Mothering in a Modern World*, contact Nature's First Law in the Resource section in the back of this book. Be sure to ask them for a free catalog of all their great books, videos and cassettes).

Home schooling is another great way to bring up your children naturally. If you are able to do it, I highly recommend it. Home schooling is the only natural way for a child to grow and learn. You cannot expect your child to learn about nature in an unnatural room being taught by someone who they don't know. In the wild, you don't see any animals leave their young babies to another animal to be taught. They always teach their young themselves. Even if you are not able to home school your children, you should take them out on the weekends and teach them about nature and the natural things in life. If you want your child to be 100% natural, do not push away all the beautiful things nature has to offer. You should learn to enjoy those same beautiful things with your child. Parents and their children, living peacefully and happily in nature, living a 100% natural lifestyle, is as natural and beautiful as it gets! Giving to your child the gifts of nature and health is a legacy you can leave for the future, today.

To become natural in an unnatural world,
enjoy the natural beauty of nature.

8 | RAW KNOWLEDGE

Interviews

The eating of natural foods in their raw form has taken place since the beginning of time. First, it was the dinosaurs. Millions of years later it was the cavemen. The first mention, in the Bible, of humans eating raw fruits was about Adam and Eve. It is not a new philosophy. Only since the discovery of fire, did humans start to cook their food.

"If you looked at a clock and compared it to how long humans have been eating cooked food since the beginning of time, it would come out to about 5 seconds."

Today the idea of eating food cooked is a very normal practice. Unfortunately, so are the diseases of modern man. It is no mystery what happened. Until humans decide to get back to nature, we will continue to suffer from diseases. Fortunately, many people have not been taken in by the crazy idea of eating our food cooked.

There is much information available today about the raw food movement in this country and abroad. Some of this information goes all the way back to the early 1800's.

Today, there are many people around who have been eating raw foods for many years. I am very fortunate to have met many of these pioneers and they have all helped me on my own road to THE RAW LIFE. I have taken several of the interviews I have completed over the past years and put them into this book to help you as well. All of them are with pioneers who have succeeded at attaining a RAW LIFE.

There are many different ways to achieve ultimate health and a RAW LIFE. However, all of the people I interviewed had one thing in common, which is that they realized the value and benefits of a raw food diet. They have all lived it and felt true health. Their information will help you to do the same. Avoid getting confused if one person interviewed did something one way and another person interviewed was dead against it. Read all, learn, and do what works for you! No two people are in the same place at the same time, so you should make adjustments to go with your lifestyle. No one knows your body better than you; and no one walked in their shoes but them. They did what they did and they succeeded at it. This should be your final goal. To succeed and become a champion. You will not agree with all of them. Do what you believe and what works for you.

No school could ever teach you what these following interviews can. It would take you years to gather all this information. In the past, there was very little information available about how to get your body back to nature. Back then, you had to learn through trial and error. The people that did make the change back to being as natural as they possibly could, did so with very little information. They did not have the Internet and there was very little published literature available but they still managed to make the transition. You can learn much from their trials and errors. Use what worked for them and stay away from what failed.

182

Today there is so much information, and it is so accessible. At a time when so many people are moving further and further away from nature, these pioneers are now helping us to get back to where we belong. We have so much to learn and they have so much information to give. If you want to be natural, it is wise to learn from someone who is natural.

Here are several interviews with long-time raw-food eaters, who offer priceless information. Learning from them will help you stay a champion. Learn and live it.

"A truly educated person is he who can instantly apply to his best advantage the lessons learnt through a lifetime."
— Morris Krok

"Listen to a wise man and become wiser."

— Morris Krok

Stan Glaser

The first interview is with Stan Glaser. Stan owns Glaser Farms in Florida (See info at the back of this book). I have met Stan several times and spent many hours talking with him. I have spoken to many raw-fooders over the years and if I had to pick the one person with whom most of their concepts and ideas I agreed with, it would be Stan. I find his approach to the RAW LIFE simple and to the point. Personally, I find my own raw life taking the same road as Stan's. I hope it continues that way because I find him and his lifestyle amazing. Stan is a true legend!

How long have you been eating a diet of raw foods and what made you get into it?

I started eating a raw food diet in 1975. I have been doing this now for about 23 years. I got into it for spiritual reasons. When I started 23 years ago, no one was there to teach me what to do or how to do it. I had to develop the diet myself. I had to teach myself what to eat and what not to eat. I've learned many things over the years from trial and error. Sometimes when I really would get into trouble, there was nobody to ask. I just had to go deep inside and find the inner wisdom. Today it is different. There is so much wisdom and there is so much information out there for anybody with an interest to learn.

What are some of the things you have learned that will help people succeed in eating a 100% raw-food diet?

To start off, I think it is very important to keep a day by day journal. I wish I'd have kept one, because I have been doing this for such a long time and have been through so much. To look back, it would have helped me to see how far I had come. If I ever had a question from the past, I could have just checked my journal and read my notes. So I think that is very important to have.

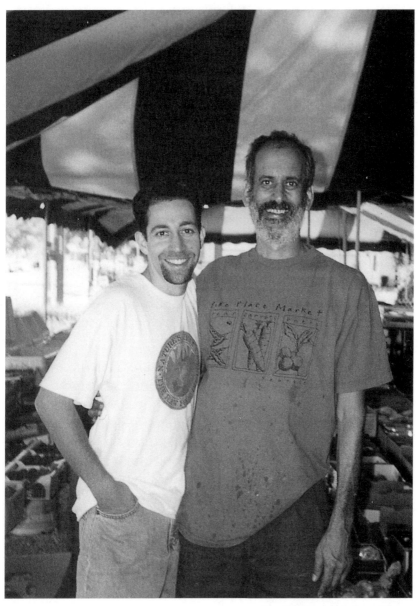

Paul Nison and Stan Glaser

Also when you eat raw foods, you have to be careful, especially if you start to shy away from eating seeds and nuts.

You also have to make sure the foods you do eat are very well grown, because what you could be getting is just water, not even clean water. You have to be careful to make sure you eat good organic food.

I would also recommend eating seaweeds. They are important considering the environment that we live in today.

Check with people who have succeeded at eating a raw diet. Learn from them as much as you can.

Stay focused. It is very easy to get involved with a philosophy that will screw you up after awhile.

Be aware that you have body parts, like teeth, that do not respond very well to changes of diet. They do not change as easily as other parts of your body and sometimes you could get in trouble with that. Be able to respond to the changes of your body and be honest with yourself.

Try not to get involved with little side trips or concepts. Try to define what you are doing in a real way and then go ahead and do it. Then watch your body and don't be freaked out by changes. Remember your body is going to have to rebuild every problem it has ever had. You are going to get pains here and there. You're going to go through many things. It might take you a very long time to straighten out all of the problems that you have created over many years. You just have to be patient.

Do not become involved in eating raw foods for the wrong reasons. If you get involved with eating raw foods to lose weight, you will lose weight, but then there would be no reason to do it anymore. If you get involved to impress people or to do this or do that, it will not work. You have to have the right reason. I think the right reason is to be in the right place in the world and to be relating to everything in the right way. That's the reason that you should eat the food that has been put here as food, and it will also help what the plant you are eating to propagate.

What is your average daily diet like?

I don't really have a basic daily diet. I try to eat once or twice a day. I eat a lot of avocados. I have really been eating a lot of seaweeds for some time now. I eat many different varieties of seaweeds. I also like bananas and I also eat some greens. There are just so many foods that it is hard to say. I just eat what I am in the mood for at that time.

How is your health and energy, how much sleep do you get, and how much daily sleep is necessary?

I am doing the job now of about five people, so I guess it is good. I could get along with very little sleep. I would rather sleep around eight hours, but being on the raw diet, I could get along with four or five for six days a week, I do rest one day a week.

Do you think four or five hours is healthy?

I do not. I think we should be able to sleep as much as our body tells us to sleep. The problem is work. I chose to do what I am doing right now. Before I was involved with this job, when I was about 26, I traveled and studied for about fifteen years. At that time I was able to sleep when I wanted to and when my body told me to. I think that is how it should always be. Right now I sometimes want to rest during the day, but because of work I can't do that. I feel the same way about food. We should eat what our bodies are craving when we are craving it, because our bodies need it. So we should do our best to sleep when we are tired because our bodies need that also. If I could get five minutes here or there to lay down I would feel better, but if our job does not let us, I don't think that is very natural.

What is your favorite food?

I like to think about it the same way as thinking of people—kind of like who is your favorite person. The answer is, whoever is really cool at that time. I would say the same thing about food. I am into whatever is available within the limits that I allow myself to eat. I get into all kinds of foods, as long as they are well-grown and well-matured. All good food is like a gift from God.

Of all the different foods, do you think any one stands out as the most important?

I do not think I could single out just one food. All foods that are natural are important for our bodies. When people first get involved eating just natural foods, they program their internal computer with the taste of a certain food. At that point and onwards, your body will tell you if that is the food you should be eating. You don't need anything written on the outside or any vitamin contents. All of that stuff is given to you in an intuitive way just by eating the food and registering it within your internal computer. You can't say any one food is best, because then you will wind up overeating that one kind of food. If that happens, you will wind up being allergic to it after a while. What you should do is basically be open to all of the foods that you consider natural and just eat what your body computer is telling you to eat by your cravings.

Many people have trouble dealing with weight loss on a raw diet. What is your opinion about this and have you been able to maintain your weight throughout the years?

People have concepts of what they should look like, and what a healthy person looks like. A wise man once said, there should be a portrait of a healthy person in a museum so people know what they are talking about. In many cases what people perceive as muscular and healthy is not the case at all. This is something that is available in the flush of youth. As you get older, what was once considered health becomes very detrimental later on.

As for my weight, I just let my body reach its own level. For example, before I started eating natural (I'm around 6'1) my weight was up to 210lbs. I have gotten all the way down to 129lbs. At present, I am at a fairly reasonable 165-170lbs. This is the weight I seem to stay at regardless of what I do.

What is your opinion about exercise on the raw diet?

People could get away with a lot by just eating raw foods. They could live in the worst city, not exercise and still survive on a raw diet. The body was made to exercise. Not necessarily strenuous exercise, that will hurt the body. That is not what I am talking about when I say exercise. What I mean is stretching the body the right way and doing yoga. These exercises are excellent for the body. Doing some aerobic exercise to get your lungs moving is also great. It shouldn't be strenuous exercise like people you see jogging in the street with all of that pain and suffering. Everything that you do should make sense to you. When you eat, you shouldn't eat something that doesn't taste good to you just because you think it is good for your body. The same goes for exercise: to do any exercise in any way that feels bad to you and is uncomfortable, it isn't healthy. Everything that you approach should be a joy. That is the direction that you want to go, but definitely exercise. I personally do not exercise that much, but that is because I get exercise in my daily work. I load trucks and lift boxes. If I wasn't doing that, I would be sure to exercise more often. I like to stretch or do yoga exercises every night. I think it is very important to include this into your life.

I am going to mention some topics. Tell me your opinion on them:

Sea vegetables

I would say that seaweed would be the one thing that would insure you of being well mineralized. They are very important considering the environment that most of us live in today. There are many different kinds of seaweed. They are all good but some are cooked. As far as I understand, Arame and Hijiki are tenderized. Make sure you get them wild, harvested, and sun dried. They are the best kind to get, and your body will do best with them.

Nuts & Seeds

They are a good transitional food. Soaked, they are a little easier to digest, but a diet with any kind of seed products is going to be a problem over time.

Grains

Same situation as with nuts.

Fruitarianism

It is a nice fantasy. Fruitarianism is a word that people could pronounce and use. People kind of flock to it because there is no real name for what people should really be eating, raw fruits and green leaves as an ideal diet. I don't think fruitarianism works in the long run.

Sprouts

A good transitional food to a real state of a perfect diet. They are raw and for most people it would be a very good thing for them to eat. If you get to the highest ranges of what we really should eat, greens and fruit, then sprouts are something that interrupts the cycle of the plant that you are eating.

Natural Hygiene

Those guys were really good. They wrote a lot of nice books. They have a lot of good information and brought the diet to a nice place considering that they were doctors a long time ago. It was probably easier for doctors to do that at that time. I think it would be harder to do it today. I give them a lot of credit. I learned many things from them.

Supplements

There is no such thing on a real diet as a supplement. A supplement is just a misnomer, because there is no such thing. You should eat what you need and that should be your food. Anything that is added on to that is not really food and it should not be put into the human body.

Eating Seasonally

It is good if you could do it. Most people do not stay in just one place forever. If you travel from a cold place to a warm place during the winter, what should you do if you were eating seasonally? Should you continue to eat the same way or not? Even though you were not in the same climate, your body would still be on the time of the place that you were at. We also live in heated places. Sometimes we do not go outside for long periods of time, so seasonal eating is not as valid as it used to be.

Fasting

In the past, people would go on a fast more for spiritual reasons than for health. Today people mainly do it to lose weight. It is something that people spend a lot of energy and effort doing for a short period of time. Most of the time when they come back from the fast, they have exhausted all of their willpower on the fast. They wind up eating worse or at least the same as they did before. When this happens, the cells that they just hollowed out on the fast, just fill up again with the same stuff. Unless you can incorporate it like eating once a day, kind of a daily fast for a long period of time, it really doesn't make much sense. It takes a long time to change the cells of the body and for them to transform. I suggest to just get behind a steady diet of eating the right thing, day by day and you will do better in the long run, instead of trying to fast periodically and wasting yourself trying to do that.

Food combining on a 100% raw foods and is it necessary?

If you are eating the right things and you vibe into what you are eating, you could eat whatever you want in any combination. I think food combining is an attempt to simplify something that is a little bit more complicated. I think it works more when you are eating meats, starches and things like that. But when you are eating raw foods, especially when you are getting close to eating just fruits and greens, then food combining as it is written in the books is invalid.

Overeating

I think constant eating or overeating is a problem people have. They are putting undigested food on top of half-digested food. I think that is more of a problem for a raw food eater than food combining. Today people eat more for impulse than for when they really need to, just because our society likes to eat. I think that this is a big problem.

Wild Foods

Great! All foods should be wild.

Spirituality

I think a reason many people don't have much success on raw food diets is because they are not used to living on that level of lightness or that level of energy. People really don't get energy from food. They get energy from the cosmos. It is your God-given gift. This is why if you fast a little bit you have more energy than you know what to do with. You can't even sleep. So what we are doing most of our lives is using most of our energy to digest food. Not necessarily getting energy from the food. As you eat lighter and lighter, your body can process more easily without using all of its resources. When this happens, you will start to experience lots of energy. This new found energy does not feel grounded to the normal person. This is when it is very important to have a spiritual context. I think spirituality at its best is teaching your body and mind how to deal with this infinite energy. If not, you won't feel good, or as I say, grounded, and you are going to wind up eating heavier foods to use the energy again. I think it is very important to have success with the raw diet. You have to learn to combine the diet with spirituality—that deals with infinity. This is what spirituality is, and it is what we as human beings could do. We could really learn and understand infinity. I would highly recommend to anyone who wants to make progress to find somebody that can teach them more about these other techniques.

What are your thoughts about the life cycle in food?

The way to deal with food and understand food is to know that there is food that is here for us to eat and that it is here for no other reason. In other words, we are put here in a situation by a creative force that loves everything. The only reason we feel pain is because we are in the wrong place at the wrong time. We are eating the wrong foods. We are getting involved with animals and taking their lives. When you eat the body of an animal, it is not what was meant to be. The animal really wants its body to grow and live. We are using them for food, even though they were not put here as food for us. There is so much food that has been put here for us. The easy thing to understand is a fruit. The fruit drops all its seeds under a tree. It can't grow all those young trees under that one tree. It needs an agent to pick up the fruit, to eat the fruit and when it is finished, it will throw the seeds far away from the tree so the seeds can grow into new trees. Or the seeds will process through the body in an indigestible form and be spread. So in other words you are helping the tree and the tree is helping you. It is a beautiful situation, as opposed to when you get involved with eating meats. It's even worse, because you are getting in the way of a being growing. So the ideal way for us to eat would be where everything is aided by everything else. Where food is aided by eating. This is the situation I understand we can have with all things.

Do you have anything else you would like to mention to help people. Any final thoughts?

I think people have to decide what they are doing and what they want to do. They have to be convinced. First they have to convince their mind that what they are doing is what they have to do. They have to define the parameters of what they want in the total spectrum of foods they are going to eat. They have to get that really well defined. Then just go for it.

Watch and observe your body. Observe the cravings. Play with it so that you can deal with those cravings. Just watch the process and don't get freaked out by weight and by pains coming and going. You can massage different parts of your body to get rid of that. There are all kinds of things you can do, but you have to allow the process to happen.

Aris La Tham

Aris is one of the most famous raw food chef in the world today. He has been eating raw foods and preparing them for many years. His food tastes great and his knowledge about the lifestyle just blows my mind. I am so thankful Aris took the time to share his knowledge with me, so I could pass it along to you.

How many years have you been eating a 100% raw food diet and why did you start?

I have been on a 100% raw-food diet for 22 years. I started for analytical reasons, reading about it and out of curiosity. Applying it and seeing that it really works has kept me doing it.

Is there any one person who has inspired or helped you when you were first learning about the raw food lifestyle?

I did not have any direct influence or inspiration from any one individual. I grew up in a time where I could not physically go and meet someone who was eating 100% raw foods. It was not until I met Dick Gregory and Viktoras Kulvinskas that I was able to do that. Before meeting them, my greatest influences were through reading. Reading material from Dick Gregory, Viktoras Kulvinskas, Arnold Ehret, Dr. Norman Walker, Dr. Lust, Dr. Richter and his wife and Hilton Hotema. All of their writings have had a tremendous influence on me. There are quite a few good authors who have written about being natural and eating raw foods. Studying the information and understanding them, then putting it into practical use, helped me realize that it really works. I was able to maintain myself on it, but it really was a total lifestyle shift from what I was used to at that time.

If you had to give just one piece of advice to staying on a 100% raw-food diet successfully, what would that advice be?

I think the most important is to try to avoid tasting any cooked food. If a person eats cooked food, it will stimulate their desire for more.

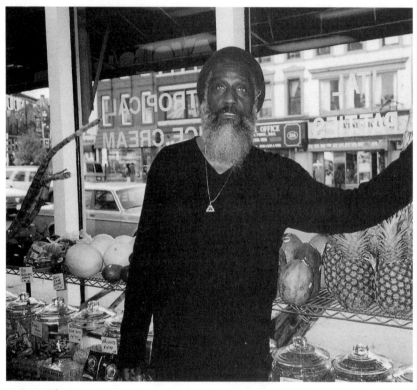

Aris La Tham

What are some other important points that will help people succeed with being natural and eating 100% raw foods?

Having support is very important. Forming a support group, support from your family and friends or anywhere else you can find it is very important. Having this support to reinforce the lifestyle is very critical, rather than hanging out with people who are on the opposite end of the scale. Misery loves company and all people influence each other some way or another. We have to make sure we are very careful about that.

Also stay informed. Keep reading and keep getting updated information all of the time. Talk to people and learn.

You must also keep an open mind and realize that reaching a 100% live food lifestyle is not instantaneous. There is a transitional period that most of us have to go through. It depends on the individual and the individual's body how to go about this transitional period. I have even seen some people go from a total omnivorous diet to a live food diet overnight, and they have been able to support it. Much of it begins in the mind and it ends there also. You must be careful and pay attention to your relationship with your mind.

What are some pitfalls that people just starting out on a 100% raw-food diet should watch out for?

Just as I said before, introducing any kind of hot food into your system is going to trigger stimulation by your body to demand more. I would also highly recommend not smoking any marijuana. Many people who are just starting a 100% raw diet claim to be natural. But there is nothing natural about smoking marijuana, it is cooked and all cooked substances are poisonous to the body. Getting high from marijuana also stimulates your appetite for cooked unnatural foods. I don't believe anyone who gets high and then tells me that they are 100% raw natural eaters. Getting high is unnatural and if you do get high, it will cause you to crave and to eat unnatural cooked foods. It is a chemical reaction of the body. This is a serious pitfall for people today who want to be hip and get high. If you are smoking marijuana and you don't want to stop, then a 100% natural life is not for you. A diet of live raw foods, the way nature intended it to be, will give you a permanent high. Another pitfall to watch out for is association and relationships with certain people. You need reinforcement and support. You have to really stand your ground, because people are going to ridicule you, they are going to do all kinds of things to discourage and discredit you.

So any cooked foods will stimulate feelings for raw fooders to get off of a 100% raw-food diet. Would you say the same thing about frozen foods? Are they as bad and unnatural as cooked foods?

With any extreme temperature in foods that you ingest, the body has to bring it to body temperature. Whether it is hot food or cold food. Your body cannot get very hot foods past its windpipe. The body has to cool it down right there. The same thing happens with frozen foods. The body has to warm it up right there. In doing that the body has to produce many enzymes. So it zaps your energy after awhile. For these reasons I would be careful with frozen foods just as I would be with hot food. Frozen raw foods are not as detrimental as hot foods, because the enzymes are still somewhat available to you, as opposed to the cooked hot foods where they are not.

What about frozen foods that are frozen and then re-warmed to room temperature before they are eaten?

It would still be relatively safe, but it is not natural. That would not be part of a live food lifestyle. Any frozen food in any form would not be part of it. It would be a safe transition for people who feel for whatever reason that they cannot eat 100% raw natural foods. Remember though, fresh is always best, there is really no other way.

A big discouragement to many people is that when they attempt to eat a 100% raw-food diet, they lose weight they feel they cannot afford to lose. What is your advice for people who doubt the raw diet because of this?

There is no question about it, most people are going to lose weight on a live food diet, because your body cannot build in a dirty house. We live in a society that has created some serious problems for people when it comes to weight, because practically everyone is overweight. So we seem to be normal because so many of us are like that, but the body should be light and should not be overweight.

What is your opinion about exercise? Do you exercise?

Yes, I do exercise, but not rigorous extensive exercise. I mostly jog or swim. Also, I lift many fruit boxes and other stuff everyday, so I get my exercise naturally. One of the things that I find is, it is good to do something just for the sake of doing it, but when you do it for a cause it can become very mechanical. It is like people in ancient times. In order for them to get their food, they had to climb a tree. They would get their exercise from climbing the trees. To have to go to a gym and actually put yourself through that is fine for the modern lifestyle if that is the best that you can do. I think we should try to achieve these things through living and just being. We should let it happen naturally and get our exercise in our daily natural living.

Another big discouragement people have are problems with their teeth. Do you have any advice on this?

I find the sugar in certain fruits definitely harms the teeth, especially citrus fruits that are not ripe on the tree. One of the problems we have today is that many of the fruits eaten today are picked green and unripe. Unripe fruits are too acidic for our bodies and our teeth. When we eat unripe fruit, this acid wears down the enamel on our teeth. People really need to be careful with this.

What is your average daily diet like?

I am eating about 70 to 80 percent fruits right now. Not just sweet fruits, also the vegetable fruits and the non-starchy fruits as well. The protein fruits also. I have mostly liquids in the morning and some juicy fruits, such as citrus, pineapple or something like that to open up my system and cleanse it. Then in the latter part of the day I start eating more dense fruits that have less moisture. Closer to dinner time I will eat more non-sugary fruits such as avocados, olives, coconut, tomatoes, cucumbers, bell peppers and so forth. Sometimes I may add some lettuce, celery or some light vegetables that are easy to digest. I usually enjoy eating a mono diet, foods by themselves rather than having them mixed with other foods. I try to stay as much as possible on light foods that are high in moisture.

What is your favorite food?

If I had a favorite food I would not eat anything else but that one food. I would strictly be on a mono diet of that food. I truly enjoy papayas. Sometimes I like to go on a papaya fast for 14 days. I do this about once a year. If it is not done with papaya, I do it with mangos. I also love young coconut water. This really makes my skin shine. I like fruits much more than I do vegetables. They just appear more natural to me.

Do you think that there is one food that is most important?

No, I do not think any one is most important. I think we have to have many different foods in different combinations and in ample varieties in order to satisfy our nutritional needs. Not only our nutritional needs, but also to satisfy the desire to keep eating healthy. Out of all the many foods that are available to man today, I think the one that might be healthiest on a natural basis is the papaya, because of its digestive enzymes. The way it breaks things down very easily, it is the best tenderizer around. They even use it to tenderize meat. It is the best food that you could eat for enzymes. Good organic grapes with their seeds are also excellent. They cleanse the body and build it at the same time. There is no other food that could realistically do that.

How important are green leafy vegetables are to have in the diet?

I do not feel that they are super important once your system is clean and your body is no longer full of toxins. For people to really enjoy leafy green vegetables and get the maximum benefit out of them, I think it would be best to have them in a juice form. I feel it is good in a juice form, but not absolutely necessary if you are living the way nature intended us to live.

How is your health and energy?

It is great. I am 51 and compared to other men much younger than me, I have much more energy. I have not been diagnosed with any medical conditions. I have been a vegetarian for 28 years and eating 100% live foods for 22 years. I do not have any problems with deficiencies or anything like that. I may have a B-12 deficiency but so what, am I supposed to be crying because I am lacking vitamin B-12? That is not an issue for me. When you really analyze things like that, of all the B-12 eaten in animal products, the body only utilizes about 5% of it. Beyond that, our bodies have the capability of producing our own vitamin B-12 as long as our system is clean.

How much sleep do you get, and how much do you think is necessary for people to get?

I average about five to six hours a night. I think it is necessary to get as much as you can. It is best to go to bed, lay down, go to sleep and just get up when you wake up. If you are getting up by an alarm clock, you are shocking your system. If this is happening, you will not know if you are getting the required amount of sleep for your body. If you do this, you are programming your body to work on less sleep than it needs. To keep this up is like whipping your body to keep going. It depends on the individual. I find that the more cooked foods you eat, the more toxins you put into your body, and the more foods that you eat are difficult to digest, then the more sleep you will need. The reason for this is because this kind of food will not really get processed until you are sleeping. Then you miss out on the cleansing effect and the building effect of those foods because the time your body should take to do that, it is instead busy processing and digesting. That is why if you eat those types of food you get tired. You find that after a big, heavy cooked meal loaded with starches and proteins you go right to sleep. That kind of food just knocks you out because the body has to produce so many digestive enzymes. On a live food diet, it is not easy to get to sleep because the body has so much extra energy. However, when I do get to sleep, I try to enjoy it and I try to sleep until I wake up.

I am going to mention various topics. Please share your opinion on them.

Nuts & Seeds

They are fine. They are great for getting protein. They should be soaked to remove the enzyme inhibitors, so that the digestive enzymes that break down the protein are active to actually break it down. Otherwise, they will not digest properly and they could cause health challenges for the body.

Grains

Like all starches, grains are not a necessary food, since the body has to convert them into sugar in order for it to be utilized. There is already enough sugar in fruit for the body. The body does not need any extra. I would keep grains to a minimum. If you do choose to eat grains, always sprout them and process them as much as possible without actually cooking them.

Sea vegetables

Seaweed's are great for the body. You can't get anything better for the minerals and trace minerals they contain. They also add an extra flavor to foods. Seaweeds are a food that I try to eat everyday. I would rather have at least a little amount than none at all.

Fruitarianism

The nature of human beings is that of a fruitarian. By nature we are more closely related to all of the frugivious animals. When you look at our anatomical structure, the digestive juices, so forth and so on. We give birth just like the frugivorous animals and we don't have many similarities to the carnivores or herbivore animals. If you really look deeply into those facts, you would see what I am saying is true. Even if you want to consider the scripture in the Bible that states "Behold, for I have given to you the seed-yielding trees." Right there it says that your food should actually yield a seed. Food that has the ability to reproduce itself without humans tending it. The only food that can do that is fruit. Fruit trees are actually food factories. For the most part, you don't have to do anything to them and they will just keep throwing fruits at you, year in and year out. Make sure when we are talking about fruits that you do not limit yourself to just the sweet fruits. There is more to fruit than just sugar. Avocados, bell peppers, tomatoes, cucumbers, squashes, eggplant and so forth are also all great and very important fruits. Remember anything that comes to you with a seed is a fruit.

Sprouts

Sprouts are great but they are a little overrated. I feel they are overrated because there is no other way to really eat the things that you sprout. I see sprouts as a group of different types of live foods one could eat. I would not emphasize eating too many sprouts, as I said, the foods that you eat sprouted can't be eaten healthfully without sprouting them. For this reason you should have sprouts only if you are going to eat foods that need to be sprouted and could not be eaten healthfully in their natural form.

Natural Hygiene

Natural Hygiene is a great dietary movement that started quite some time ago. It was actually a revolt by Christians against the Standard American Diet (SAD). It was a Christian revolution. It has held up very well throughout all these years. Natural Hygiene consists of some very strong practices in terms of getting as close as possible to a mono diet without mixing too many foods. Unfortunately, Natural Hygiene still includes some cooked food in their dietary regimen, and they do not soak their nuts before eating them. These are two things that they could actually learn from modern advances in the live food diet. That would be very helpful to them.

Supplements

Supplements are not necessary. If you have to supplement your diet with something else, then your diet is deficient, so why even bother with supplements, improve your diet!

Eating Seasonally

Eating seasonally is a reality if you live in a certain type of environment. However, if you are living in a place like New York where only apples and maybe some berries are available in the winter, what are people supposed to do? Should they fast the whole season? Eating seasonally is something that was brought forward in a very big way by the macrobiotic movement. But what they advocate in their system, they really do not support. They eat a lot of brown rice and brown rice does not grow anywhere close to New York. Brown rice is also a seasonal food, but people who are on a macrobiotic diet eat it all year anyway. Beans are also a seasonal food that they eat all year no matter what the season is. These are some reasons that I do not support the idea that eating seasonally is important. Also, when it comes to the climate and climate issues for example, should we or should we not eat tropical foods in the winter? I don't think that holds either, because even though people live in a temperate climate, they still live a tropical lifestyle. They are in cars, buses and trains, they wear underwear, longjohn's, masks, gloves and all kinds of other stuff to keep their bodies in a tropic like environment. People are not living naked and rolling in the snow like bears do. You can get the sunshine through your food like fruits if there is no sunshine where you live. Also, when people are in their houses, they turn up the heat very high so it feels like they are in the tropics. So even though we live in a temperate environment in ways, we are still living a tropical lifestyle. For this reason, tropical foods are just as good for us in the winter as they are for us in the summer.

Fasting

Fasting is our safety valve. It is something that people have been doing since the beginning of time. We do it spontaneously and involuntarily without even realizing it. Every time we go to sleep at night we actually go on a fast. The system just shuts down and digestion ceases. When this happens, elimination takes over. People defeat the purpose of this daily fast by breaking it incorrectly. They forget about what breakfast really means. Today people call it breakfast. People forget that it should actually be a breaking of a fast. Besides fasting once a day while we are sleeping, we should fast once a week for a thirty-six hour period. I recommend this so the body can truly get a rest. Also because it gives its organs a chance to rejuvenate and to recuperate—to get all of your organs strong again, so when they do go back to work they are fit and ready to go. Also, I recommend taking it a little further and incorporating a seasonal fast, once on the solstice and once on the equinox. Fast during this time for a three-day period. Fasting at these times is recommended because during this time the body automatically eliminates. The tissues, organs and the intestinal track eliminate many toxins at these times. That is why many people end up with the flu and all these other things. It is really just a mass cleansing that is taking place universally.

Is food combining on a 100% raw food diet necessary?

Not the way it is available to us today. We have to remember that today's food combining laws have been derived from the initial studies on cats that were done by Dr. Pottenger. We also have to keep in mind that it is based on cooked foods and that the enzymes have been destroyed in the foods. I find with food combining that you definitely could flex beyond the rules of the charts that are available today if you are eating 100% live foods. I think it is much more important to look how foods grow and the amount of moisture that's in them. I would classify foods based on that. If you really look at the food combination charts you see how they are grouped. The high moisture fruits are in a group of their own, the melons are 99% moisture, the acid tasting fruits are about 90% moisture, the pulpy fruits and the sub acid fruits have less moisture and your sweet fruits have even less. So we should really look at the moisture level of the fruits and also how they grow. The higher in altitude the food grows, the more cleansing and electrical it is. The lower in altitude the food grows, the more magnetic it is and the more building they are. That is the starches, the root vegetables and the grains. These dense foods are lower in moisture. So of course we naturally can keep these apart. There is also a little more fine-tuning that we could do to these charts to make them more user-friendly for the live food diet.

Wild Foods

Wild foods are the best for our bodies. They are the greatest. The way we are now, we have moved into a collision course with nature by hybridizing our foods. We are at the mercy of agriculture, businesses and all of those crazy food giants who are just producing food for profit, not for people. So we end up with many toxins in our foods which are manufactured and processed. If we could get more wild foods, we could get more back into life and nature. That is the way to go, eating as much wild food as possible is best.

Is there anything that you would like to add?

Yes, It is the life in the food that really nourishes the body. That is what counts. It is not the food in your life that matters at all. If you don't realize that, you just end up eating up all these empty calories and all of these loaded foods that really don't have much value to our bodies. These foods leave behind too much toxic waste in your system. Anyone truly interested in maintaining a live food lifestyle, really needs to keep in mind that initially the body is going to detoxify. When this happens you are going to lose weight because the body does not build in a dirty house. This holds true for people who want to get well also. Live natural foods will clean that house. If you have any medical conditions that modern medicine says are incurable, live foods will help you get rid of them. I think it is important to eat live foods as a lifestyle and not wait until you get sick. This is one thing that I find I was blessed with. When I started on a live food lifestyle, I did not come to it because I was sick, I came into it from an eater's point of view. In this way, I was able to develop a cuisine that crossed boundaries, so you don't even have to be a vegetarian to enjoy the live foods that I have created. I have developed them in a way that it will heal you just as well. I have added some energy, some flavor, some taste and some vibration to it. That makes it possible for all people, not just sick people to enjoy eating it. Unfortunately, most of the people that are on a raw food diet or who have expanded on it, first started eating live foods because they were ill. Those people then developed a diet that is very cleansing, very pure, very clean and perfect, but of course with that very bland, very tasteless and very

207

basic. It is important for mainstream people who are not ill to enjoy and develop an appetite for live food. Unfortunately, people who are ill go on these cleansing, therapeutic diets and once they feel better they go right back to their old ways. We need to really look at things in a more practical way and be able to give people certain things that can help them maintain and support a lifestyle of live food over a long period of time. Not just to get well but to stay well, to be happy, to be healthy and to multiply.

"People are my nourishment. They nourish my soul. Without them, I would be deprived of nourishment."

—Aris La Tham

Gil Jacobs

If you don't believe in the power of THE RAW LIFE, meet Gil and he will change your thinking. His dedication to getting the word out about the raw lifestyle is amazing. I am so happy there are people like Gil in this world. He makes a big difference. After I interviewed Gil I could not wait to edit his interview and review what we spoke about. He brought up many great topics.

How many years have you been on a raw food diet and what got you into it?

I have been doing this now for 18 years. I got into it because I was deadly ill. I went through a dramatic experience when I was 21. I got very self-destructive because of it. Afterwards, I realized that I did not want to die. I was in the hospital very close to the end and a good friend of mine came in and said I should get into alternative healing. He brought me some books to read. One thing led to another and I fell into the raw-food diet, deep tissue cleansing and juicing. Those three things healed me. So, it has been 18 years now and I am still doing them.

Who have been some people who have inspired you to do this and is there one person who has inspired you the most?

I am a friend of Viktoras Kulvinskas, the author of *Survival in the 21st Century*. I differ with some of his views now, but at the beginning of my healing, he was a driving force. He is totally into it for the work. He has a great vibe to him. He was a great source, but the biggest influence for me was someone I have never met. If I could go back in time to meet one human being, it would be this guy. Arnold Ehert, author of *The Mucusless Diet Healing System*. I go back to his concepts continually. Fred Bisci from New York has been another very big influence on me. Norman Walker's books are also very important.

What do you think are some of the most important things you have learned to help you successfully stay on this diet?

I think the thing people need to know is that they have to walk before they can run. There is no doubt about it. The raw-food diet is the natural diet of human beings. Given the desire, everyone has the ability to do it. The blood type system, the ten food group system, they're all wrong. The raw-food diet is for everyone, but to get to the point where you can do it 100% is the tricky part. People have to realize that the more toxic they are when they start, the slower and more easily they have to go. If they go too fast they can literally loosen up too much poison and they can get very sick. I think the biggest concept is for people to assess where they are when starting the raw food diet. If the raw-food diet at the beginning is a little too rough, they should ease into it. Do it 50-50, and let their body detox. I honestly believe within a year everyone can be doing a 100% raw-food diet, but I think you have to get to that point where you work the system on a tissue cleanse before you just jump into it. This is especially true if you were ill at the beginning.

Is there one big pitfall people should one watch out for when starting a raw food diet?

I think it sounds funny but people ask me, "how do I know if it is working?" All you have to do is look in the toilet. If your body is efficiently eliminating toxins, you will never have a pitfall. But if elimination slows down, bones start aching, pimples come, sleep gets restless, and the breath becomes bad. What is happening is the raw food is loosening up more poison than the body is letting go. That is the major pitfall. People have to know what to do when that comes up. If they do not, it can make the diet look bad.

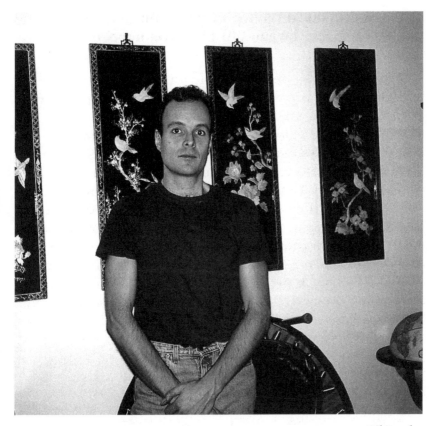

Gil Jacobs

Two big common pitfalls most people have are problems with weight loss and problems with their teeth. Can you comment on both of these?

I had both of those problems badly. The sicker the person is when they start, (sadly, it is almost a guarantee) the more problems the teeth are going to give them. One reason is that they have mercury in them. When you have mercury fillings and you get into a radical raw diet you have a contrast there. You have a toxic material, mercury, which gets hit by a cleanser. When that happens, the teeth are going to revolt. Also, the

211

body tends to release poisonous acid through the head cavity and the teeth are going to suffer because of this. If the bowels and cleansing rate can keep up, you can keep teeth problem to a minimum.

Weight-loss—I think people have to understand it is your body healing. They have to avoid associating diseases like cancer and AIDS with weight-loss. Too many people do this. If you have a big dirty sponge and it is dirty with water and crap, the only way you clean it is to squeeze. When you squeeze the sponge, it temporarily gets small. That is cell contraction. When you finish the squeezing and you let go, it is going to puff back up a little. What people need to do is be calm and easy with the fact that they are going to get very thin if they stick with this. People have to understand that thinness is the cell contraction. It is the healing. If they live through it and they allow themselves to come back, they get a taste of immortality. You cannot heal if you do not get thin.

On the subject of weight-loss, will all people doing a 100% raw food diet become too skinny? Is it possible for someone to become overweight on a 100% raw-food diet?

I think that if someone stays overweight, something is wrong. Probably what they are doing wrong is trying to use a raw-food diet to create a body that modern man thinks is appealing. Understand that you are not going to win Mr. Olympian on a raw-food diet. If a person is trying to jam raw goat's milk cheese, raw egg yolks and eleven avocados a day into their body to maintain a body weight, they do not yet understand the principle of under-eating. The living food lifestye is about living on light, and air, with a little bit of food. If a person is very large, and staying very large, for me, they are not healing, and they are not going to achieve health and longevity. It just does not work like that.

On the subject of teeth, for people with mercury fillings, do you suggest getting them removed? If so, replaced with what? On the other hand, do you suggest waiting for them to fall out naturally?

In my own case, I am waiting for them to come out naturally, which sometimes happens on the raw diet. If you get the mercury fillings out, you are going to prevent much of the clash between cleansing fruit sugars and poisonous mercury. It is an expensive thing but I think everyone, if possible, should try to get the mercury out.

What do you suggest if the mercury fillings come out? What do you recommend replacing them with?

The only thing I know that is available right now is porcelain. Some people use gold, but then again you are putting a metal in the body. I am not sure this is a very good idea. The porcelain is less toxic. Since people into raw foods are very strong, the slight toxicity of the porcelain is not going to be an issue. You deal with more toxins walking pass a bus. The carbon dioxide from a bus is going to be worse than porcelain fillings. Therefore, I think that is the best bet.

I am going to mention various topics. Please share your opinion on them.

Nuts & Seeds

Raw nuts and seeds in theory work well. Especially at the beginning, if people are coming off meat, eggs, milk, and cheese. Their body is going to need the stimulation, otherwise it is going to cleanse too quickly and they will get ill. In addition, the cleansing response will drive them crazy. What people have to understand is that nuts and seeds are some of the most concentrated foods on the planet. Do not eat a pound of nuts. Only eat a handful. That should be the limit. Nuts and seeds are not ideal, but if they are eating a 90% raw food diet, this is great and they will probably live a long time. If people

213

want to achieve the best health, I think after a couple of years, they should look to eliminate nuts and seeds, or at least soak them twelve hours before eating them. If you soak them, some of them will at least germinate, making them easier for the body to digest. People have to understand that it is not about being perfect. However, if you do eat them, you should not snack on them. This is another thing that people are doing and that is wrong. You cannot put nuts in the body and then ten minutes later eat a salad. A raw fooder should think of nuts the same way a person eating the "Standard American Diet" thinks of steak—as the main part of a meal.

Grains

I think in terms of the ideal. People should definitely use them the first year and then if they're really into trying to live according to health principles, they should limit grain-eating, or better yet, give them up completely. This is because grains are mucous-forming. If you are coming off a totally Standard American diet, whole grains are going to be an important transition food for at least six months. This is because it is relatively better than what they were eating beforehand. However, what you want to understand is that grains are not ideal. They are not human food. If your goal is to get to the highest level of health, you should gradually, over the course of a year try to eliminate grains. If you are happy with a 50-50 diet of raw salad and cooked grains, that is fine. You are probably going to live a very long time. But you are going to see, when you get into your eighties, your health may start going down-hill.

Is the Fruitarian diet complete, or do you feel some greens are necessary?

In the 20th century, I definitely feel a greens are necesary. Eating only fruit in any big city is just not going to work. This is true for a number of reasons: One, getting enough high quality fruit is difficult. Two, we are all products of weakened heredity. Our parents were probably unhealthy, and their parents probably ate terribly too. For ten generations, we have been coming from a lineage of bad eaters. We are not born with the genetic inheritance that the first people on the planet were born with. There is no doubt about it. At the beginning of time, fruitarianism was the perfect diet. However, I really don't know if our bodies are now equipped to eat only fruit. Three, when you throw in the pollution, radiation from computers, poisonous fumes from wall-to-wall carpeting, tight clothing, walking on asphalt, florescent lighting, make-up, deodorant, and all the other nonsense, the body needs a healing element. Chlorophyll from greens is the greatest healing element.

Hybrid Fruits

I think in a perfect world we should not eat them. However, a hybrid fruit is still better than an organic grain, an avocado or a raw nut.

Sprouts

Alfalfa sprouts just do not taste good enough to me to be an everyday food. I honestly believe if food is an everyday food, it has to taste good. I do think for medicinal reasons they are good juiced, but there is a lot of research that says those little brown covers on them are carcinogenic. I certainly don't have the time to pick them off. I stay away from them because they do not make a good intestinal broom. If people are eating just alfalfa sprouts and buckwheat lettuce, they do not eliminate well, because those things do not sweep. However, if you are 100% clean, you can eat them. If you want to juice them, I think they are great, but as for eating them, I do not know. I would still rather eat lettuce. The other thing with sprouts, if they should be eaten everyday, they would be out there and they are not. They have to be man made; they require work.

That tells me they are not for healing. Once you are 100% clean, you do not need them.

How important is a 100% raw food diet? Is anything less just as good?

It is great as a goal, but I don't think that you should take anybody and put them on a 100% raw-food diet. It could be a death sentence because too much poison is going to loosen up at the beginning. The idea of being into 100% raw food is excellent, but you cannot grasp it like a religion or a cause. For different people, the amount of time it is going to take to get there will vary. If it is a healthy 21-year-old basketball player out of college on a good diet already who wants to get into an all-raw diet, it might take him two months. However, if a 55-year-old accountant with a belly hanging over his belt wants to get into an all-raw diet, it will take him much longer. I think he should have as a goal that he is going to get into it, and maybe take two years after he starts, to go all raw. He should go 50-50, half raw and half-cooked, when starting the raw diet. Then his next goal should be eliminating all the animal food. His next goal after that should be three-quarters raw. In about two years, I think he might be ready. However, for someone in that condition to jump in feet first, I think it is going to give us all a bad name. I think the raw diet is the diet of man and I think everybody into health should have it as a goal. However, they should not rush into it. Yet, they should not think it makes them less of a healing person if they are not 100% raw.

Do you believe everyone could eat a 100% raw-food diet after they have cleaned out?

Most definitely. Everyone has the body to eat a 100% raw food diet once they are clean. One thing that upsets me are books that come out from these so-called healers. They are saying things like it depends on your blood, it depends on where you are born, there are 10 types of human beings and it depends on which one you are. That is so upsetting. What it depends on is how clean your body is and how long it will take to get clean. Everyone, I believe, can get there. In the perfect human state, I think we should all eat 100% raw-food diet.

Do you think the concepts of Natural Hygiene are the best concepts to follow?

I think physically yes. The problem I have with some of the people that have started the Natural Hygiene lifestyle is that they do not account for inherited energy. When you read Shelton's books, he keeps going back to the Garden of Eden, and that is my big issue with the natural hygienist. They say don't do colonics because they are not natural, you don't have to make juices because our bodies don't have juicers attached to them, don't do this and that because that is not the way people did it at the beginning of time. What they are not getting is that the sperm and the egg that creates a human being carry the toxicity of the mother and father. We have 10 generations of poisoned people. We do not have the capacity to live in accordance to the perfect natural law unless we cleanse and prepare our bodies. That is what colonics, juicing, massages and full spectrum bulbs are for. If you do not incorporate varius healing methods to rehabilitate from the effects of generations of poor lifestyle, then the natural hygienist lifestyle can kill you. You cannot jump in overnight. At the beginning, a certain amount of unnatural activity has to take place to get people there. That is my only difference.

Supplements

I think they are nonsense. Arnold Ehret had a phrase he used at the beginning of many sentences. He says, "the entire trash of human dietetics," and then he goes on to finish the sentence. It is a lot of nonsense, because it is a belief. I call people who are into supplements "putter-inners". They think we get better because of what we put in. They think that illness comes from what we are missing. If you go to the average chiropractor or the average nutritionist, this is what they do. They do some type of wacky muscle test, spit test, hair test, or urine test. Then they come back and they say, you're not getting enough riboflavin, you're not getting enough vitamin B-6, you're not getting enough pantothenic acid and then they give supplements to you. That has nothing to do with health. The key is, the thing people are not understanding, is the reason you are missing these things is because all the bad food you have put in your body from birth has burned them out of your system. The crap in your body, the carbonic gas is sticking in your cells, eating away the riboflavin that you were born with. We were all born with these things. It eats away all the things that are missing. The way to get yourself better is not to add them in pill form. Remove the poison that is sticking in your cells. When you do that, your body will assimilate the nutrients it needs from foods. Supplements to me are a total waste. They are useless. I will not change my opinion about this. One thing though. There is a difference between concentrated food and supplements. When I talk about supplements, I am talking about vitamin A, vitamin B, vitamin C. Spirulina and certain algaes I think are great because they are just foods put into powder form. That is different than taking a B-6 supplement. So there is a difference between a concentrated chlorophyll food in powder form and vitamin/mineral supplements.

Eating Seasonally

Personally, I do not eat honeydew melons in February. The reason is that they are coming from places that don't have very good reputations in how they grow and handle the food. I tell people to try not to eat food from some Latin American countries because radiation levels are very high. However, if somebody snapped their fingers and gave me Malaysian fruit in the middle of February, I am going to eat it. I don't have a problem with that. I do have a problem with where it comes from. I don't buy the macrobiotic concept that we cannot eat papayas in February. If I can get them from the right place, I would eat them all year.

Fasting—Juice vs. Water Fasting

I think fasting is good if people do it in an unattached way and in the absence of ego. One of my problems again with people that get heavily into hygiene is, they use fasting as if it is a championship belt. They say things like "I did a forty day water fast, did you?" There is too much ego attached to the length of time people fast. I think little fasts are excellent. It calms the body and at the same time it allows a certain level of toxicity to release, especially if done over ten days in conjunction with colonics and enemas. If it is not, and a person loosens up many poisons in a fast, (which they will) it stays in the body and it reabsorbs into the blood. You can end up with broken bones (which I have seen). You can also end up with pimples as big as golf balls, your hair comes out, and your teeth fall out. Many hygienists tell people to just grin and bare it. That is nonsense. If those people were doing colonics, all the poisons being released would come out instead of being reabsorbed. They are going to feel as fit as a fiddle and not going to end up looking like they are dying. The one catch though is, once you do colonics or enemas on a fast, you must get chlorophyll. You must also get high level fruit sugar. You should not do a long water fast if you are not going to do cleansing methods, because if enzymes do not go back, you can get extremely fatigued and sick. I do not like long 30-day fasts because of the way people come out of it. I never met anyone who has done it without bingeing afterwards. It seems to me that, many people that do very long fasts also have problems with very long binges. I think the reason is if you loosen up a lot of old heaviness and you don't get it out, the body becomes aware of it. It looks to feed that craving. Therefore, if people are going to do long fasts, I think they have to get into colonics everyday, at least enemas. Long fasts in the absence of colonic and enemas to me are like jumping without a safety net.

What about a fruit juice diet or any juice fasting?

Juice fasting is OK to do longer periods of time. I think that if you are healthy you can go on a fruit juice fast. If you are unhealthy and you want to do some fruit juice fasting, that is fine. Again, the very second you get a bad symptom that means it is time to do a colonic or an enema. This is because the only thing that makes people weak and sick during a fast, is not lack of nutrients, it is old poison, which has loosened up in the colon, and it must come out.

What is your opinion about a 24 hour fast on juice or water?

I think that is great. I wish I had the discipline to do it. I think we should all fast one day a week for life. It does much good. If people are into colonics or enemas, the best time to do it is the morning after you have done a 24-hour fast. I have seen it do wonderful things for people. During the 24-hour fast is also a good time for people to relax, meditate and be at ease. I think short fasts are excellent.

Food combining on a 100% raw food diet. Do you think it is necessary?

I think you should still combine foods optimally. When you are eating 100% raw, since you have eliminated starches and you have eliminated dense proteins, there are less combination pitfalls. Norman Walker believes we can eat all fruits with vegetables. It does not work for me. I believe what the hygienist say here, that romaine lettuce and celery or all lettuce and celery mix with fruits. The idea of eating spinach and peaches does not even sound or feel right. We should eat nuts and seeds with citrus fruits or vegetables. I do not particularly like sub acid or sweet fruits with nuts and seeds. Unless you put

15 or 20 minutes in between them. But if you are mixing it all in a bowl, nuts and seeds go better with citrus fruits and vegetables. I don't really know where other combinations come in because we're not eating starches. As for fats, if people are going to use extra virgin olive oil, it should never be used with nuts, seeds or avocados as that is a terrible mix. I cannot think of any other combination issues. One important thing is the order of the food we eat. I think there is not enough emphasis on it.

You mean like sequential eating?

Yes. You should not eat an apple after an avocado but you can certainly eat them together or eat the apple first. You should not eat a raw salad after a durian but you can certainly eat the raw salad first. The thing people need to remember is to eat light foods before heavy foods, and after heavy food is eaten take three hours and eat nothing. You do not want to eat a salad an hour after an avocado because it will ferment in the stomach and cause problems. So yes, the sequence of eating is something which should be paid more attention to by health seekers.

Why did you say it was good to eat nuts and citrus fruits together?

Nuts and citrus fruits works because low sugar fruits, especially ones with acid, will help break down protein. Therefore, for a healthy person, I recommend this. For someone who is healing with this diet, I wouldn't recommend it. For a healthy person, two citrus fruits and a handful of almonds will work fine. Oranges, pineapples, green apples, and strawberries mix well with nuts and seeds. For someone who is sick, they should just eat nuts and seeds soaked, and they should just eat them with just a salad. In this way, it is easier to digest.

Exercise

I think it is necessary. Really hard exertion, if you're into weightlifting, with a weight as heavy as you can handle, good form, and low repetition, is a great way to release gas pressure from the body. If you are a raw foodist, this really works. If you get a little headache, go to a flat bench and do about three reps to the maximum, or do a couple of other lifts, like the beginning of the Olympic lift. All of a sudden, you get this lightness and sense of well being. Your headache will go away. The reason is the body is releasing blood gasses through the skin. It really works. I think weightlifting is a great thing. It takes a bum rap because a lot of health oriented people associate weightlifting with the bodybuilding lifestyle. The bodybuilding lifestyle is truly the death lifestyle. All that excess protein and amino acids are deadly. Weightlifting has nothing to do with bodybuilding. You can be a raw fooder and workout with weights. I think yoga, weightlifting, trampoline (especially magnificent for lymph drainage) dry brush massaging, walking, and deep breathing are all outstanding. One of the problems I have with some raw food people is they get so light and airy from the cleanness, they sit around too much. There is too much non-activity going on. I do not think that is a good thing.

Wild foods

If a person is sick, I think wild foods do a lot of good. For me, as long as you are healthy, no one should eat anything on a regular basis that does not taste good to them. If someone really likes bitter tasting foods, then they should be an everyday food for that person and they should eat it. What I find is some people are eating these bitter leaves, hating it and eating it everyday because they think it is good for them. That's no good.

Hair loss and the raw food diet

I am so against people that go for hair analysis. The body knows what is most important. There is something called Herrings Law of Cure that speaks about this. The most important organs in the body are the ones in the belly. The ones behind the belly button, the colon, the kidneys, the spleen, the liver, the lungs, the small intestine, the stomach, the pancreas, the prostate, and the uterus. The body worries about these organs first. It is going to feed them first. Then it will come up to the heart, the lungs, and the thyroid. When it gets all the vital organs, it will then go to the extremities. When people lose hair, it means there is something imperfect, but it does not mean they are toxic. The body knows hair is less important so it feeds the hair last. Therefore, when a guy starts losing his hair, yeah it means his cells are not 100% clean, but it does not mean he is dying. It does not mean he is toxic at all. Hair loss simply means that the body does not have enough chi-energy to get to the hair. When you get into raw food, what often happens is you lose all your hair because the system is going to get rid of the old. It has too much protein and it is too acidic. It is going to give you new hair. Seven years ago, I had very little hair. I was almost bald. Now I have a full head of hair. What is going to happen is you are going to lose it and then it is going to come back. It happens with women also. It is funny, they scream "I'm losing my hair." What the body is doing is it is getting rid of hair that is too acidic and it is going to grow new hair. That is what hair loss is all about on a raw food diet.

Just as in the process of detoxification?

Totally, it is out with the old, in with the new.

Can a person's hair color change from gray back to its original color?

Oh, sure. Many people have. Viktoras Kulvinskas is one of them. Washing hair with wheatgrass will do that because it gets into the follicles. However, even through just improved diet and cleansing, hair will grow back and often changes color.

Reversing poor eyesight naturally on a raw diet

We inherit certain traits from our family lineage, not just from our parents, but from our entire past heredity line. If you look at my left middle toe, see how much taller it is than the big one. That means I was born with a weak stomach. All the cleansing in the world is not going to make my toe shrink. This is because I inherited a weak stomach. I can make my stomach very strong, but that particular thing is not going to change. I have been wearing eyeglasses since I was four. When I was around 17 years old, I was as blind as a bat. As you can see, now my eyeglasses are much thinner. My eyesight has gotten much better. I can walk around without them and I can drive without them, but I still need them. I firmly believe if I keep doing this work, keep fasting, doing colonics and living "in the light," I am eventually going to throw away my eyeglasses. Nevertheless, I think it is important for people not to get attached to perfection. To just take it easy and look at the fact you are doing great. Look at the rest of the world and look where you are. Love the fact that you are doing much better than in the past. You should take joy in your successes and not fixate on your imperfections.

What is your opinion about the natural eye exercises, especially the Bates method? Do you think they work in helping to improve eyesight?

If you have the time to do these eye exercises and you are really into getting rid of your eyeglasses, yes, it works. I have seen people do it.

Even for people who have inherited poor eyesight?

Yeah, what you will see is you can improve, and as time goes on, and you continue to cleanse the body, your eyesight will come around.

Can you talk a little about fruits and the difference between seeded and pitted fruit?

All fruits are good for the body. The perfect human fruits are the seeded fruits. Five are "top of the line": figs, apples, watermelon, papayas, and grapes. Those are the perfect human foods. Perfect 100% with the seeds in them. When you get to foods with pits, you are getting to foods (if you look at the flesh of pit fruits) that are a little bit denser. This does not mean they are not good. They are excellent. Physiologically, a mango or a nectarine is not as perfect as a fig. When people get really into this you may notice if you make a lunch of a bunch of mangos, you might get a little sleepy. It sits in the body a bit longer than a bunch of figs. It is just an interesting little point. One thing I do recommend is to be careful if you combine the two. If you are eating a bunch of mangos, do not eat it with a bunch of apples. Keep the pits with the pits and the seeds with the seeds. That tends to work best.

So what you are saying is that fruits with seeds are more cleansing then fruits with pits?

Yes, they definitely are, especially for deep tissue cleansing. That is why when you look at many of the books that deal with a specific fruit cleanse, there is the watermelon fast, the grapefruit cure, the grape cure. No one has ever done a peach cure, and there is no plum cure.

What is your age, height and weight? Would you talk about how your weight has changed over the years?

I am 42, around 5'10, and right now I am about 138 pounds. People are going to hear "138" and go "huh?" What they have to understand is when cells are clean, a low weight looks a lot better on a raw fooder, than a low weight looks on someone whose cells are dirty. If you looked at the average American man who is 5'11 and 138, he is going to look like he is dying. When you are into this lifestyle, it is a whole different look. The cells have what are called "cellular integrity". They are clean. The reason people are lighter in weight is because when a cell is healthy, it is not holding excess waste products inside. It is not holding gas so it is very tight and compact so you do not carry a lot of weight. People eating a raw food diet look much better naked than they looked dressed. The reason is you put clothing on and your cells are not puffy. They do not fill the clothing. People will say "you look like a skeleton" or "you look like a wire hanger with clothing on you." Once you take off your shirt, they leave you alone. They say wow, the guy looks good. I always tell men when you get into the raw-food lifestyle if you are getting thin, forget about how you look in a formal suit. Instead, look at yourself in a bathing suit. You are going to look much better. When I got sick, my weight was down to 108 pounds. When I got into doing the raw food diet, I went down to about a 100 pounds. I kept doing the diet because I knew it worked. My family wanted to incarcerate me. I kept doing it, did the colonics and the juicing. I juiced a ton. I did psyllium seed, bentonite, and more colonics. I went up to 140 pounds, and I was not eating any heavier. The reason I went up to 140 pounds is that my body was clean enough to do so. The body knows that it should not be 100 pounds. No human being should be 5'11 and 100 pounds, but while it is healing, it is contracting. It is squeezing out poison. Like squeezing a dirty sponge. It makes you stay 100 pounds until you are clean enough to bounce back. I did not change a thing yet over one summer I went from 109 to 142, and I did not add heavier foods. It is a vitally important concept for AIDS and cancer people to grasp. They are going to get skinny. It does not mean they are dying. It means they are getting healthy. My weight has gone down to 100 pounds and up to the low 140's. Now it is 138 pounds.

What is the most that you ever weighed?

I once weighed 207 pounds. I was a bodybuilder when I was 19. I did two muscle shows. I used to eat a dozen eggs a day, chop meat, and two whole turkeys a day.

Have you ever been medically diagnosed with any disease or illness?

I've had hepatitis, diverticulitis, fatty acid deficiency in the colon, anemia, almost pernicious anemia and irritable bowel syndrome. Doctors thought I was anorexic. I also had some acute kidney disease. I do not exactly know what they called it. In addition, I was totally impotent for seven years. I never went to a shrink or took any wild herb. Just from healing, I now have children. That is why I am so dedicated to this lifestyle.

Do you eat a 100% raw-food diet, if so for how long?

I just did three weeks of eating 100% raw foods. Because there are certain things emotionally that are not what I want in my life, it puts me through a lot. When emotional things hit me, I sometimes eat cooked vegan food. Right now, I eat about one cooked vegan meal a week. On the average, I guess I eat about three cooked meals a month. I know I should not do it, but I do it for emotional reasons. However, it is not physically the right thing for me to do. My body is physically clean enough to be 100% raw, but the fact is I am human. I use cooked food as a comfort thing. I do not beat myself up about it. I know eventually I will be 100% raw—I am very close.

What is your average daily diet like and how often do you eat?

My work is somewhat hectic, so this throws my schedule out of whack. If I have a day when I am not working, I will wake up and I will not take in anything, not even water, until I feel the need. Usually what happens is about 1:00 PM I will make a quart of lettuce juice. Then I will go for an exercise workout. When I come back, I eat about two pounds of juicy fruit. After that, maybe four hours later, I will juice another head of lettuce and I will probably eat some romaine lettuce and celery with some nuts and dried fruit. Sometimes I have just nuts or maybe just an avocado. I might even have another bunch of juicy fruit. If it is a day I am eating cooked food, I always make sure I eat a huge amount of green leaves. No one who is heavily into health should ever eat cooked food in the absence of raw green leaves.

What is your favorite food?

When I'm in the United States, my favorite food is fresh black mission figs. I wish the season were longer. I could eat them by the truck load. My second favorite would be good Haitian mangos. My third choice would be good persimmons. In Thailand, my favorite foods are papayas, pineapples, jackfruit and sapodillas, which are amazing! Notice that in Thailand, there's not as many pit fruits, there's mostly seed fruits. The only pit fruits are mangos and durians. Anything that is ripe is great!

Of all the foods, which do you think is most important?

If I had baby coconuts available all year round I would throw away my juicer. I would just drink coconut water and have one fruit meal a day.

What are your views on sleep and energy?

During sleep, the kidneys clean the blood. It is like natural blood dialysis. This is the reason people get dark rings under the eyes, because that is the sign of an overworked kidney. The kidneys function best during sleep. If the average person does not get sleep, that means their kidneys did not work well. They get colon or kidney rings. The beauty of being inwardly clean is that four of five hours sleep is sufficient. Especially when you are eating light. Needing less sleep gives more time to be productive. When people have insomnia, what that means is that they are so toxic that their body does not even have the ability to get into a sleep-state. If they are sleeping 7, 8 or 9 hours, that means they are OK. They are in that middle level of health. Their kidneys are still filtering blood. What will happen with many people who get into raw food is that they sleep a lot at the beginning. That is fine because the kidneys are doing major blood cleansing on old blood gases. You will see as you stay into this for years, the sleeping time will go down, down, down. When you are clean enough to sleep 4 hours, you will sleep 4 hours. If you need 7 or 8 that is fine. Do not worry about it or take it as a sign that there is something wrong with you.

Would you say good rest is the same as sleep or are they two completely different things?

Rest is important for the mind but sleep and rest are two different things. The kidneys will not function to the degree during rest that they do during sleep.

How much sleep do you get on the average every night? What do you think is necessary for the average person?

I think when people first start eating raw foods, they should allow themselves at least 7 hours sleep. This is because when they go through detox, they are going to require this much sleep. Right now, if I get 4 1/2 hours I feel great. If I get five, I am super. However, if I eat a cooked meal, that night I need closer to six. This is because the body needs more time to clean the blood. If I am doing all raw or I am fasting and it is the summer, 4 hours is sufficient for days on end.

What mental changes have you noticed on this diet?

My mind is very clear. I can carry five conversations at once. I can pick up, process, and remember things very quickly. It is the accuracy, the sharpness, and the ability to re-call information. The ability to keep track. I have about 600 clients and I could tell them things they told me six months ago. There is no doubt about it. Sluggish brain and dull witted-ness, is all dirt, waste, and gas in the body. It is all about diet. I guarantee you, any human being, I do not care how dull wit-ted they are, if they get into this lifestyle, in 5 years they're going to be as sharp as a tack. I will take that to the grave.

What if someone was born with something like Down Syndrome? Could they ever be normal?

If you notice, a lot of Down Syndrome children eat, eat and eat. That is because toxicity wants toxicity. If you put Down Syndrome children on a raw-food diet and gave them colonics and enemas, I guarantee in a couple of years they can be 75 % normal. Probably never 100%, though, because their genetic inheritance has been damaged them at birth and that is a shame. Congenital childhood diseases come from poor heredity, not just by the mother and father but even further back in time. The Pygmies are fruitarian. There are no Down Syndrome pygmies. There are no Pygmies born with child birth defects. There are no Pygmies dying in their 20's and 30's of degenerative diseases.

For people who are not familiar with the Pygmies who are they?

They are the tribal people in New Guinea and Africa. There is a great book called *The Forest People* which speaks about the Pygmies.

What is your opinion about interpersonal relationships and how has your opinion about them changed since being on a raw food diet?

I am a very flexible person. I make demands on no one. It is not my style. I let everybody do their thing. If you really want a harmonious relationship and you are really into this, I think you have to find someone who is at least a vegan. Someone who is at least very health conscious, does not smoke or drink. They must at least honor the power of the raw-food diet. They may not be doing it 100%, but if they think it is a crock and they think you are a fanatic, and they love you anyway, sadly, I really do not think it is going to work. I have told people, if you are really into this, try to find someone at least who recognizes the brilliance and the beauty of the lifestyle. If you do, eventually they will come around. If their laughing at you lovingly thinking you are just a very cute lunatic, it is not going to work.

Thanks for sharing your time and knowledge. Is there anything you would like to add?

Yes, I'd like to emphasize how powerful the effect diet is on good and evil and ethical living. If the entire world's population got into raw food, cleansing gradually and easily without getting obsessed, and also got into meditation, and if we did this for a couple of generations, we could loosen our rigid concepts about money, police, passports and the military. Everyone could live in peaceful anarchy. Because when you live 100% clean, the desire to hurt, to get violent, to get angry, to be perverse, and to be selfish disappears. I honestly believe that the reason we have shrinks, the reason we need prisons and Prozac is cheeseburgers, pizza, milk and drugs. People attempt to address anti-social behavior through a psychotherapist. They really need to address the issues connected to their belly. If they cleaned out their body and learned how to eat, meditate and live with nature, I honestly believe we can have Utopia on Earth. As idealistic as it sounds, every problem on that plane, from schizophrenia to homicidal behavior, start at the level of the cells and then manifests in the mind. I think that is something raw food people need to grasp. Look at how happy and content you are. Most people can't compare to that. You are unattached to stuff, you don't need jewelry, cars and stock certificates. You don't need to go out at night to a club. Being human and just being alive becomes enough. I think that is the thing that people have to grasp. The last step is the raw food diet, fasting, colonics, meditation and sunlight. Proper feeding creates nirvana and creates a society that can do nothing but nurture itself and nurture others. That's something I'd like to create with a small group of people with the same vision.

Dr. Tim Trader

Whenever I talk to Tim Trader, I feel his energy buzzing in the air. He is doing a great job in passing on the message of THE RAW LIFE. His knowledge and background will help all that pass his way.

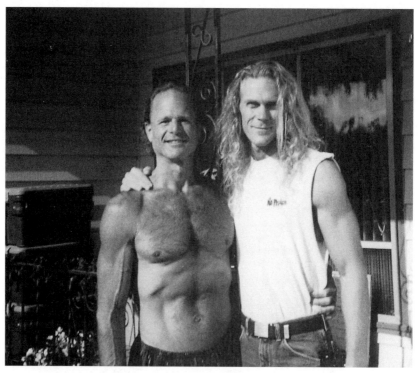

Dr. Tim Trader (right) with Dr. Doug Graham

How many years have you been on a raw-food diet and what got you into it?

I have been on the raw-food diet almost nine years. What got me into it was a life-long problem with asthma and allergies. When I was growing up, I was allergic to proteins in my own mother's milk, in cow's milk, in goat's milk and soy. Therefore, my health was poor from the start. Prior to being raw, I spent five years searching for the correct homeopathic remedies to cure my asthma, but it wasn't until I found raw hygiene was I able to actually stop my asthma attacks. I learned what was really going on with asthma; not what medicine said was going on with asthma. So I have been there almost nine years, and I have not had an asthma attack since.

Who have been some people who have inspired you on the path of health? Is there one person who has inspired you more than anyone else?

I think the real inspiration is the truth. As for people who have inspired me, there are so many. Herbert Shelton, TC Fry, Doug Graham, Ann Wigmore, Viktoras Kulvinskas as well as other well known raw fooders of the past whom have helped me to some extent. I remember TC Fry was there for me at a time when I really needed support. Doug Graham also helped me a lot. He was a kindred spirit. As for books that have inspired me, most people read *Fit for life* by Harvey and Marilyn Diamond first. I read *Superior Nutrition* by Herbert Shelton first. That book was just awesome to me. Then I read *Fit for Life*. Both of those books really inspired me when I was first getting into this. People also inspire me by watching their mistakes and understanding what is going on. I learned from Shelton who was someone who made some mistakes. He became a martyr. I do not want to be a martyr for this cause. I try hard not to be. I want to live long.

What do you feel is the most important thing you have learned on this diet and this path?

I would say common sense. Man has scientifically gone so far askew from common sense. If you get rid of addictions, get inwardly clean and pure, then following your own body wisdom, these are the greatest things. I do not see it just in food, I also see it including technology. Yet we sometimes make technology our god instead of being part of our evolution. I think common sense is the greatest thing that comes from this. It is the wisdom of nature.

What pitfalls may accompany the raw-food diet?

I see many problems with how people approach this diet. One is the term "mono diet." People decide they are going to eat only one kind of food for a very long time. I see many problems come up from this. Every once in a while I hear someone say, "I'm just going to eat oranges and nothing else." The mono diet is not the idea of just eating one thing. It means eating only one thing at a time. If you were in the wild, you would be going from orange tree to apple tree, probably getting some greens here and there along the way. That is true mono eating. Eating just one food all the time will only lead to problems and is a big pitfall. You should be aware of that. Another pitfall is being unduly influenced by others. Many people who eat just raw foods worry so much about B-12 deficiencies. I see more B-12 deficiencies in my office from meat-eaters than I have ever seen from raw-foodists. Listening to the stories about vegans not getting enough protein is another one. So many people worry about that, and they should not be worried. Another big pitfall is letting others worry you with their fears.

Two common pitfalls I find in people on the raw diet are weight loss and teeth problems. What is your opinion about these issues?

First weight-loss. Everybody is worried about weight-loss. This is because we are in a society that considers obesity as normal. Society looks at people slightly obese as healthy. We have to get over this addiction. You will lose weight on a raw-food diet, but we all have to clean house at some point. I tell most of the people who come to me with weight worries "you will gain it back I promise"—and it always comes true. Their weight may not be as much as they were before, which is OK. Second, most people I have seen who do not have mercury fillings generally do not have the teeth problems that other fruitarians or raw food eaters do. A big reason for this is that mercury increases the acidity in the mouth. That is a big reason for cavities. Some people also have problems with fillings falling out. I think that when you eat raw foods for several years, as your body becomes healthy again, your body gives you a sign that the fillings are not natural. They will eventually fall out, especially mercury fillings. They are very unnatural. In addition, many people had teeth problems long before they started eating a raw diet.

When you talk about decaying are you talking about receding gums as well?

Most of the time, I see people who brush their teeth quite a bit, and when they are fruitarian, they are still brushing their teeth heavily. Because of this, what we see as receding is not necessarily receding, but inflammation. People who lightly brush their teeth or do not brush their teeth at all seem to have very healthy gums. I think that is really the key. I think this is another fear that people have.

You suggested that mercury fillings are not natural to the body. What would you suggest replacing them with?

I am not a dentist but from what I see, porcelain seems good. I do not know all that much about the new dental materials that are available. I have heard of a new glass material that is very good and stays in for a lifetime. I am interested in finding out more about this material. Also, instead of filling teeth, sometimes having a tooth removed is the best choice. I once had a tooth removed and it is still gone. It is unfortunate but as a child, I had many teeth problems. I am still working on the teeth issue myself but I think it is getting better and better.

I am going to mention some topics. Please tell me your opinion on them.

Nuts & Seeds

Most people overdo nuts and seeds because they are so addicted to protein. Americans just eat too much protein. I think nuts and seeds can be a good part of the diet. I have heard them called "the junk food for the raw-foodist." I think that as long as you feel good after eating them, then they are OK. The big thing is to enjoy them and feel good afterwards. If you are just eating them and you do not feel good about it or do not like them, this is bad. If that is the case, just don't eat them.

Grains

I know there are some people who think that they are great. That's OK if you think that way, but for me I find I feel much better when I am not eating them, even if they are sprouted. I have a quote in Dr. Doug Graham's book, *Grain Damage* which says "I never felt better when I am not around grains" and that is the truth. I find that all grains, especially the hybrid grains, are not good choices for our bodies. I personally stay away from them and I direct most people who take my advice to stay away from them as well.

Is the Fruitarian Diet adequate in itself, or are some greens necessary?

I think that greens are valuable as long as you are not eating green foods that are toxic. Of course, some greens are toxic, such as the leaves of celery, just be careful what you eat.

So you think greens are useful in a diet? Do you think they are necessary?

Probably not 100% necessary, but I find people living in cities need them more than people who may be in the jungle.

Sprouts

I do not think sprouts are necessarily that important in the raw-food diet, however they are not something I would turn my back on either. I do not believe making a whole meal out of sprouts is ideal. I do not think we could find that many sprouts in nature to make a meal of them alone. Besides, I do not think I want a whole meal of them. They are good, but I do not think they are tasty enough for a whole meal. I like sprouts with my regular salad vegetables. I love sunflower sprouts. I have sprouts once a week or so, but I don't know if I would want to eat them day-in and day-out.

Juicing

I am not big on always juicing. I juice a little bit here and there. Dr. Norman Walker did well with juicing. He outlived most of his alternative health counterparts and, as I understand, they could not find anything wrong with him at the coroner. He juiced a lot everyday and lived to be over 100 years old. I do not condemn juicing, but I think that whole foods offers what is best for our bodies. I could sit and juice an orange in the wild so it is not necessarily unnatural. I do enjoy some juices, especially on a hot summer day, but I don't think it is the best practice in the world and the answer to all health problems as some people claim it is. In addition, with juice fasting, I think you can do nothing better than a water fast accompanied by true physiological rest. I think the healing happens much quicker this way.

The Natural Hygiene Diet concepts

There's a lot there. It is very good. I might not always agree with all of the old writings, but it is still the closest thing that I have found to the perfect diet. I follow food combining rules all the time. I think that real natural hygiene is more than just a concept of diet. I think Natural Hygiene touched many good points such as the importance of exercise and rest. However, hygienists sometimes do not give enough attention to the importance of mental poise. I think that was because they really did not understand it themselves. For the most part I follow a more hygienic diet, but I am getting more and more to calling it just a natural diet, instead of a natural hygiene diet.

Supplements

I think supplements are for people who are eating bad diets. When I was eating a bad diet I made a lot of strides personally with supplements, however, I tell everybody do not stay on supplements for the rest of their life. There are better things. Normally I get about 50 times the RDA for most nutrients except for protein. When you consider the value of organic food, I get something like 100 times the RDA in my everyday diet. Organic food is much more potent in truly absorbable vitamins and minerals than any supplements. If people ask me, I tell them you do not need vitamins, and you do not need mineral supplements. I say "change your diet instead of taking supplements." That having been said, I do not walk everybody's path, and one thing I have learned is non-judgement. I tell people who are interested what is going to work, but I cannot do it for them. If you are already eating 100% raw foods, there is no sense in taking supplements. I do not see a need for them.

Sea Vegetables

I have seen some people who do well with sea vegetables. On occasion, I eat them. I am not very big on them. I do not make them a normal part of my diet. I know some people who think that you should have kelp or dulse or something everyday. I do not agree. It is not a perfect food. Many people say sea vegetables prevent or reverse demineralization. Well, it might be high in minerals, but it also has a lot of sodium chloride in it. I would rather not have that sodium chloride in my body.

However, I do not think it is bad enough to stay completely away from sea vegetables altogether.

Garlic, onions, spices & stimulants

I will not have these foods in my diet. They really affect me, even in the smallest amount. I don't always notice it if I have had some in a meal. I don't physically feel it, but my attitude really does change. I get agitated very quickly. It has happened to me every time I eat these foods. So the old hygiene thing about staying away from spices and things like garlic I agree with 100 percent.

Eating Seasonally

It would be nice if we could, but 90% of us live in a place where it is too cold to grow anything in at least two seasons of the year, if not three. So eating seasonally is not so important or even practical.

Fasting: Water vs. Juice fasting

I already talked about juice fasting. I think water fasting is far better. I know many health professionals will recommend juice fasting instead of water fasting because it is safer. You cannot go as wrong as you can with a water fast. I think this is a matter of the health professional just being on top of it and no more. Whereas with a trained doctor or a trained hygienist, if they are monitoring that person well enough, they foresee problems before they come up. I am not necessarily talking about just monitoring the blood, which seems to be very popular these days. If you look at people, look at their skin, their blood pressure and check their urine daily, I think that you will find you get the answers to the problems before they come up. I have fasted myself many times. The longest is 21 days on just water. Dr. Doug Graham helped me with that. I have done several shorter fasts along the way. I do not fast regularly now. I don't see the need for it. If you watch an animal in the wild, they fast when they need to. I think I am at a point where my

239

body is clean enough so I do not have to do fasting regularly. If I need a fast, my body is now clean enough to tell me. I will have a cleansing period. Commonly we know this as a cold. If this happens, I will stop eating. In cases like that I usually stop eating for three days and try to get as much rest as possible. Then I start rebuilding right after that. When the cold dissipates during a fast, everything's going fine. If I am ever in an unnatural environment, I might get sick. One time I got what people would call pneumonia. I fasted for 7 days. I got rid of it and I was fine. I do a fast when I need to and not just to do a fast. I see many people just doing a fast for no reason but just to fast. A lot of people fast just one day a week. I don't see a need for that. If you are fasting for anything under 72 hours, you do not get any healing affects. You usually tear down muscles and organs to get sustenance until the body is ready to convert over to ketosis. When you do a fast long enough for your body actually to go through the whole process, that is when you really get results. For women, it sometimes takes at least 48 hours of fasting, but for men generally, who especially have not been on a raw regime, it takes 72 hours just to get into ketosis. Then the healing process is just beginning. People say they are going to fast three days a month, or seven days every six months. Some of them combine all of these together just to say they fasted, but unfortunately, without giving their body enough time to heal. I think they are tearing down more than building up their health. I think that nature has to tear down and re-build in a natural even flow. Once you have done the raw diet for some time, your body is going to tell you when to stop eating and to fast. When many of us have been on the Standard American Diet for 30 years like I have, on at least something close to the American diet, then we do need a planned fast to put us back to balance in order to clean up our palate and to rest our bodies, to get things started again. That is why I did my 21 day fast. It was great. It worked so well that I do not need to fast regularly. Now the people that I have helped with cancer and other serious diseases, sometimes they do need to do an occasional fast, but they're doing some serious cleansing because their body is really in need of it.

So are you saying it is better if you do decide to fast not to plan it ahead of time, or just fast when your body is asking for it?

When you are clean, yes that is what I am saying. When your body tells you "hey, I am overloaded here. I need to do something." Sometimes stress will tell you that also. Remember, if you're just not hungry, there is a reason for that. Your body is telling you something.

Food Combining on a 100% raw-food diet and is it necessary?

I practice food combining everyday if I'm not eating a mono meal. I keep sweet fruits together. I do not put a protein with a starch, etc. I do think it is necessary to practice food combining on a 100% raw-food diet. If anything, it is something that contributes to health. Food combining works for somebody who is having poor digestion, so why would it not work for somebody who has good digestion? The issue is not about, "if it is raw it has enzymes." If you could conserve your energy to have it later, why would you choose not to? Just eating anything haphazardly does take more energy to digest because of the different transit times of foods through the gastrointestinal tract. The human body can digest watermelon in 15 minutes, but if you eat watermelon with pecans, digestion is going to take two or more hours, depending on the amount eaten and what other things are with it. What will happen to the watermelon is it is going to ferment inside you. You will then have alcohol inside your body. Why would you want that? I think that with all the extra enzymes raw fooders are getting in their diet, they will still be so much better off than people eating cooked foods. However, they will do even better if they followed food combining rules and eat a 100% raw-food diet. It should become second nature to you. It makes a whole difference from just eating raw to being superb and eating raw.

Exercise

I know many people who eat raw foods and do not exercise. They just do not look good to me. Their body is not like something that I would expect to find someone who is eating a natural diet to look like. We find indigenous people like of the Amazon who have not been affected by western society so much. They may have a little bit of a belly to them, but for the most part these people could work most Americans to death in the first hour. They are just constantly going. I think exercise is essential, but I think it is more essential to be active. Sitting, watching TV and being a raw foodist is not necessarily what you should be doing all day. Being out and active is very natural and what our body needs. If that means swimming when you are at the beach and just having fun playing in the waves, that's exercise, but we can also call it activity.

What is your age, height and weight, and could you also talk a little about the changes your body has gone through over the years?

My age is 38. I'm six feet even. My weight is 150. I am a little low in weight now because I've not been to the gym lately. I've been working too hard. I like to be about 160. When I started eating raw foods nine years ago, I was 175. I went down to 131 pounds right away when I first went raw. I lost that weight in the first 3 months on a raw diet. I couldn't gain an ounce. Then all of a sudden I started to gain back my weight. I keep my weight up by doing exercise, usually weights and other resistance-type exercise. work. For me, weight is not a problem or an issue.

Do you eat 100% raw foods?

There have been times and places where I was not able to get raw food. Sometimes I ignored it and fasted my way through it. Sometimes I could not. I am not perfect. I will admit to it. I do not want to be perfect. It is too much responsibility. I am still working on being 100% percent, but I say I am 99.9%, so I think I have done well.

What is your typical daily diet, favorite food, and do you think there's one food that's most important?

Watermelon! There is no question about that at all. I don't think there's one food more important than another. If you want to start getting into the idea of one more important than the other, then you start getting into the idea like this food heals this and this food heals that. I would say give the body what it needs and allow the body to do the healing. So all different foods can be just as important. There is not just one food that is most important. Daily, I get one or two meals a day that are mono meals and then I usually have one a day that is kind of a mixture, but I try to keep it well-combined. I do not always get that but I do the best I can. I don't worry about the rest. As an example of my typical daily diet, let's take yesterday. I started with a quarter of a watermelon for breakfast. Then I had two 32-oz smoothies. They consisted of water, dates, and bananas. That was my lunch. Then last night I had four Fuji apples and some greens. Then afterwards I had some medjool dates.

How much sleep do you get and what do you think is necessary?

If you are waking up to an alarm clock, you're not getting enough sleep. Sometimes I sleep ten hours. On occasion, I can even sleep twelve. Generally, I get somewhere between 6 and 7 hours. Once a week I usually do wake up to an alarm clock, but I try not to make a habit out of it. Usually if I'm at my computer writing and I get into something, if it gets late and I know I have an appointment the next morning, I will set my alarm to make sure I get there. Many times, I have gone months without ever listening to an alarm and I sure like that. I think that is the best thing. I know that there are some raw foodists that say they get very good sleep on four hours and wake up bright and energetic. That is great for them. Then they are probably getting enough. They are the only ones that can truly answer that. With the stresses that I have from day-to-day, my body handles it quite well when I have enough sleep along with little meditation. Sleep is important, but I am not going to tell somebody how much they should have.

What changes have you noticed mentally on the raw diet?

I am primarily a serious person. When I was in medical school, I was so serious that I could watch a comic on stage and never laugh to a word he said. Now I get many laughs out of life. I enjoy life more. When I have had cooked foods, I wonder how people who eat cooked foods ever make it through the day because it is so much on the emotional and mental state. That is a killer by itself. Emotionally I am light. I am much more able to identify the emotions that I have and be able to talk about them. One of the things I talk a lot to people about is our society and how closed off we are. We do not explore our emotions and then we turn around and we say to our partners that you do not understand how I feel. Well, most of us do not even understand our own feelings. I think life is a vast process and I may not get everything until the end of my life, but I am so much more now than I ever was. I think that raw foods have put a real big part of that in my life.

For the record what degrees do you have?

I am a nationally board certified naturopathic medical doctor. I studied many years in school. Actually, I did a lot more school than most other doctors. I found out it did not work, so

I did the TC Fry course and I am very proud that I took it. I know there are a lot of people out there that say that's just a correspondence course and how could you say that is real. For me, it is more real than anything I have ever done that is accredited by more traditional institutions. I am proud of it and I mention it whenever I'm asked about my credentials. So those are my degrees. I think degrees do not make a person happy. I think finding truth is at least a nice stretch because truth is part of love and truth conquers fear. I think that is more important than anyone's degrees.

Is there any thing else you would like to add?

I often think about the way society is running itself now. If it keeps up, we are going to end up killing ourselves. There has to be a place to take a stand. My main stand is raw foods. Also, I'm against the medical establishment. There are more stands that may not be as important, but they are also something that I need to do to complete me. I have to really find what works in nature. There is so much we have to look in order to re-examine what is going on. Not necessarily just for us, but for future generations to be able to survive, let alone thrive.

Dr. Doug Graham

Doug Graham is one of the best speakers I have ever heard. His experience on the topic of health and athleticism surpasses all. I think Doug has lectured more than anyone around today. I would be very happy to follow his example. He has and continues to make great strides in the raw food movement, making it easier for raw fooders of today all over the world to accomplish a RAW LIFE.

How many years have you been on the raw food diet and what got you into it?

I have been on the raw diet for eighteen years. The path was long. It took me almost 10 years just to find it. I tried many dietary experiments as a high school and college athlete, looking for the foods that would support my athleticism. I slowly started making little changes, dropping meat and adding a little more grains, dropping chocolate and adding carob, dropping pasteurized milk and adding yogurt, etc. Just little changes. I had no idea what I was looking for but I just kept looking, and without external guidance. I'm sure the guidance was out there but somehow I wasn't finding it. Eventually, in college, I decided to become a vegetarian. I was vegetarian for almost 8 years and vegan for about 2 more. I don't remember ever reading anything about going raw. I became vegan after reading Dr. Herbert Shelton's "Food Combining Made Easy." Then I started reading everything I could get my hands on: Shelton, Tilden, Ehret, Wigmore, Kulvinskas, Airola, Fry, and Braunstein. I developed an insatiable appetite for information. But from vegan to raw food was an inspiration. One day the light just came on. I thought, "If raw foods were so good for me, why not just eat more of them?" Finally, I thought, "Why not eat only raw foods?" Once I was eating only raw food for a few months, I discovered there was already some literature on the topic, and more coming out. I

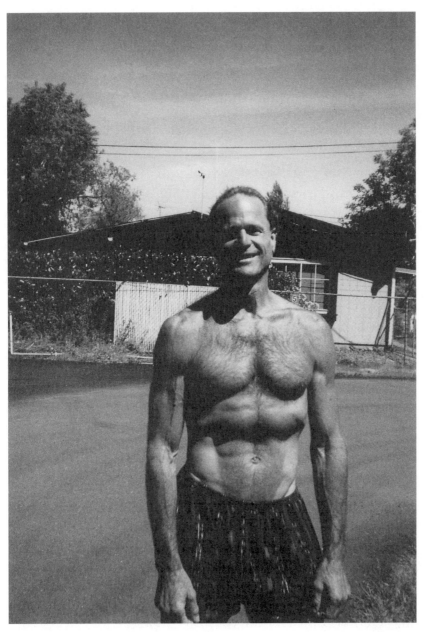

Dr. Doug Graham

was a director of a fasting retreat. I converted the fasting retreat to become an all-raw fasting retreat. As far as I knew, it
was the only one of its kind. I ran that retreat as an all-raw retreat for 10 years. For that 10-year period of time I made up all
the meals until the very last year. The result of those 9 years of
work was *The High Energy Diet Recipe Guide* a recipe book
of all raw foods, properly combined based on natural hygiene
priniciples, still the only one that exists.

How was your health when you started the diet?

I thought my health was good when I started the diet, and
although I have had my share of athletic injuries, I had gone
raw before I recognized the relationship to injury-proneness
and overall health. As a child I had quite a few health con-
cerns, especially dealing with various aspects of congestion
and allergies, but I still thought that overall my health was
very good. I was quite surprised to find my health, my attitude, my ability to stay on an even keel and my emotions, all
improved dramatically when I went raw. My temper all but
disappeared. To the greatest degree my athletic performance,
speed, strength, endurance and all of the neural connections
that involve balance, agility, quickness, and coordination dramatically improve and continue to improve at the age of 46,
after 18 years on the raw diet.

Have you ever been diagnosed with any medical disease?

I've never been diagnosed with a treatable medical condition that I'm aware of other than between the ages of 6 and
12. For those years I went to an allergist for shots every other
week. That was a horror.

Who have been some people who have inspired you the most on this path, and is there one person who has inspired you more than any other person?

I think my biggest inspiration to pursue the raw food regimen has really come from my own gardening experiences, because when I pick fruit or vegetables in my garden, it seems so right. It has always seemed so since I was a child; but growing up in New Jersey, we only gardened about 90 days a year. Now living in the Florida Keys, splitting my time between the Florida Keys and Costa Rica, I garden the whole year round. Picking fruit off the trees all-year round is always an inspiration. Humans have done this from time immemorial. This provides me with ultimate inspiration.

What are the most important things that have enabled you to be successful at eating this diet?

I think there are several key points in succeeding on a raw food regimen. These include eating when hungry, as opposed to eating for all the other reasons that people tend to eat, whether they're upset, tired, or just looking for something to do. I tend to eat when hungry and only when hungry. I also find that the more I simplify my diet, the better my energy and the better my digestion. I use this as a key tenet in diet at this point. I keep my meals as simple as I humanly can. I would say out of the 14 to 20 meals per week that I might consume at least 16 or 17 of those are mono meals. Mono meals being where I eat only one food at the sitting, like all the bananas or all the mangos that I care for. Although I know how to prepare foods, and I like to prepare raw food recipes for other people, I very rarely prepare such dishes for myself. I just eat it as it is found in nature. I also find that for success, we must include variety in our diet throughout the course of the year. This insures a nutritional well-roundedness that you simply cannot provide from any one fruit. There is no model in nature that points us towards thinking that consuming only one food on a year-round basis is to our advantage. Anthropoid apes and monkeys eat one food at a time, when hungry, until they are full, but their food choice changes with the season as availability changes. It took awhile for me, on a raw food regimen, to learn to eat enough food. As a practicing athlete, I have no problems providing myself with enough calories. But when starting out, I did have to learn to eat as much as I desired, rather than just eat a little bit of food, feel satisfied and not provide my body with enough calories. I have bumped into many people who haven't yet learned that because raw food is so much more water rich it is much less calorically dense, hence the volume we consume has to increase a bit.

What are some of the more common pitfalls that you have seen people run into on this diet?

People like to fall into a pattern. People tend to follow a religion of food, and I have not found that these people tend to succeed as raw fooders. There are people who try to live on one single food. This may work for a year or two, but eventually, on one single food, they gradually experience nutritional bankruptcy in various areas of the diet. I have also seen people attempt to live strictly and only on fruit. Although I have met a few people who have succeeded at this practice for longer periods of time, they tend to have a broader definition of fruit than the people trying to live on just oranges or just tomatoes, or just watermelon. Everyone I know (and I can think of a dozen examples off the top of my head) who has tried to live off of just one fruit has either ended up mentally insane or dead. I also think people sometimes go to a mono meal regimen, but in a way that doesn't really make sense for the human body. I met a woman one time who said she only eats mono meals. So she'll eat a pound of walnuts at one sitting, experience constipation for a week, and not know why, since she thought she was eating perfectly. So just like eating a cooked food regimen or any other regimen that people have figured out ways to follow, it still has to be done with an element of intelligence.

Two big common pitfalls are problems with teeth and weight loss. Can you comment on both of those?

Teeth are bones and people who have teeth problems

have problems with their bones. I find that people who tend to live on an over-abundance of citrus products often will run into problems with their teeth I have been told that people who pick organic citrus straight off the trees, experience much less problems with their teeth, than people who eat foods that have been picked months ago and stored, or grown with chemicals. I certainly recommend eating your fruits in season. Which means that citrus becomes a 4 or 5 month season out of the year at the most. We also have to understand that teeth problems are not restricted to raw foodists. Cooked foodists have problems with their teeth. Macrobiotic people have problems with their teeth. Vegetarians have problems with their teeth. Everybody has problems with their teeth. The thing about our teeth is that many of the problems that we experience today had their roots in our lifestyle of 5, 10 and even 20 years ago. The weakening of our teeth that has accrued in our developmental years, eventually comes to light later. It is like having a flat tire because the tire wore out. Well I mean it took 20 or 40 thousand miles for the tire to wear out. It's not just because you used it today and it went flat and you go "Oh, what did I do today to cause my tire to go flat? Today I drove a mile." Well that was not it. It is the same thing with the raw foodist or the fruitarians. I cannot honestly blame all of the tooth problems on their current lifestyle, and I do not think I would.

While we are on the subject of teeth, what do you recommend people replace their mercury fillings?

Mercury fillings are an interesting issue. Most people recognize that mercury fillings aren't healthy for us. Most of the other dental options have not been proven over any length of time either. It is my opinion that we don't really know what the heck to replace them with. We do not know if the people who are replacing their fillings are replacing them with something that is going to prove to be better than the mercury fillings. Meanwhile, in the process, you're getting another dose of exposure as the fillings are removed. If a person is having problems that they feel are related to mercury fillings, I wish them luck, but I can't say at this point that there is definitely a safer alternative.

So if a person wasn't really feeling any problems with their fillings you would recommend them not doing anything about it at this time?

Mercury fillings shrink so they will eventually drop out. But the thing about a mercury filling is that the surface area of a mercury filling is sealed and sealed very shortly after the filling was put into the mouth, and although, yes, it is still in there, it is effectively in a sealed container. There really is just as much evidence to prove that this mercury is no longer leaking into the system as there are people saying it is leaking into the system. I won't say that its a moot point, and I certainly would not say they're good for anyone. The best is healthy teeth, short of that, we have to live with what we have got.

Now could you comment on weight-loss?

Weight-loss is an interesting topic. In America and throughout the westernized world, what we find is that people in general have two qualities that are almost universal. They are over-fat and under-muscled. As people change to become vegetarians, they very often lose a great deal of this fat. As people change to become vegans, they very often lose more of the fat, and lose even more when they become raw foodists. This happens because of the relatively low caloric density of produce and people not being used to eating the volume required to insure caloric sufficiency. Also, raw foodists generally experience an increased sense of energy, are more active, and this leads to an increased caloric requirement. We often see that raw foodists end up losing a great deal of their body fat. This has to do not only with the areas I mentioned but also because of a lowered toxin ingestion and lowered fat consumption. So there are many reasons why people end up losing body fat. What's interesting is that most of them lose their body fat down to 15% or 10% body fat. Some men lose down to as low as into single digit body fat levels. This is viewed as not normal by society because in society the typical American has between a 30 to 50% body fat level or higher. So when we see someone down around 10% body fat, they look exceptionally thin. However, if we look at a greyhound, a racehorse or almost any animal in the wild that is slick and fit, we know that they have a very low body fat level. In fact, these low body fats should be considered normal and healthy. The higher body fats should be considered as abnormal. I do not want to sound judgmental, but in my opinion, these higher body fats, not the person but the body fat, should be considered abnormal, ugly, unhealthy and not supportive of good environmental, ecological use of our world. It is definitely unhealthy for the individual person. When a person loses body fat, it becomes instantly apparent that they still are suffering from the second condition that is endemic to people in the western world, which is low body muscle. If we look at most people, they look to be of a fairly good physique until we strip the fat off of them. Then we find out, gosh, they are terribly thin. They're distressingly thin, and this distressingly thin appearance is primarily due to the fact that in our western world we have developed machines and mechanical helpers to allow us to avoid any and all strenuous efforts on our behalf. We have can openers and cars, bicycles and trains and carts to roll our luggage around. Heaven forbid anybody should break a sweat during the course of their day. Effort is out and labor-saving devices are in. We are crippling ourselves with labor-saving devices. If we look at athletes, we see the beauty of an athletic body. These people have low body fat generally, and a beautiful level of body muscle. If anyone wishes to aspire to that, all they have to do is what the athletes do and they will get the same results. There are no foods that cause muscle growth and just because a person loses fat, they will be of low in muscle until they put in the effort required to gain that muscle.

I am going to mention some topics. Please tell me your opinion on them.

Nuts & Seeds

I think nuts and seeds are certainly part of the natural food of man, in their whole, fresh, raw state. However, I think that most people, certainly when they transition to a raw food diet, tend to overeat on them for several years or more. I would caution them to not overeat. Also, it's important to become aware of some of the symptoms of overeating these foods: souring in the stomach, bowel movements that come out sour, constipation, foul gas or an increase in body odor. All of these are almost immediate signs of possible overeating of protein-dense foods. A good way to think about it is this: if I were to give you a sunflower and say "Eat all the sunflower seeds you want, just start opening them up one at a time." You would probably open some and say they're good, but you wouldn't eat a pound of sunflower seeds. If you sit under a cashew tree and start eating cashew nuts, the same thing is true. I mean there is only one cashew per apple and it is a slow process to open them. In fact, you may just eat the fruit and plant the nut, that is what I always do. Macadamia nuts are equally slow to open using a couple of rocks and opening them one at a time. Any nut that you have to open one at a time is a painstaking process. It reminds us that if you have the time to sit under a tree for an hour or two, it's still unlikely that you would eat more than a handful of nuts on any given day. You would get full or tired of the opening process long before you overate.

Sea vegetables

Pond scum! I have never looked at seaweed as food. I have eaten it a few times, though. All I have ever tasted is salt. I know it is edible but I have never been at the beach, looked at seaweed, and said, "Ah, now that looks like food." I know it's edible and I know it's a very mineral and protein-rich food. I caution people about consuming too much protein. I see no need for that, and no advantage to consuming sea vegetables.

Wild Foods

I'm all in favor of eating wild foods. Wild foods tend to be higher in vitamins. They tend to be fresher, and they tend to be higher in minerals, coenzymes, enzymes, phyto-nutrients and other essential nutrients. I think that developing an awareness of the foods that grow in the wild is an asset for anyone. I think it's great to be able to pick at least some of your greens wild and as many of your fruits in the wild, as you can is great. I love the rich flavors that tend to accompany these foods.

Grains

I see no place in the human diet for grains. In fact, very few creatures on the planet consume grains as a first choice. There are some birds that eat grains, but they won't feed it to their young. I believe that any food that must be cooked in order to be consumed should be shunned. Any food that must be cooked in order to be consumed simply does not belong in the human diet. Depending on which authority you believe, we have between a 5 to 10 million year track record of success on planet earth as human beings, *without* the consumption of grains. We have only experimented with grains in the last one tenth of one percent of our time on this planet, and I believe it has proven to be an unsuccessful experiment. All we have seen during that time is a period of rapid and dramatic health decay. Again, I see no place for grains in the human diet. In fact, if you were in a very large field of ripe grains and grains were the only food available to you, you would starve before you could ever get out of that field. I look at grains as a blight on the planet earth. The sole goal of the typical farmer growing grains is to prevent all other life from growing in that field. He cuts down all the trees and he uses insecticides, pesticides, fungicides and herbicides to keep the birds and other life out. He creates a blight. The growing of grains is totally unnecessary. We can feed two and one half people on fruits and vegetables on the same amount of land that would enable us to feed only one person on grains.

Is fruitarianism sufficient in itself, or are some greens necessary in the diet?

I believe that the natural diet of human beings—at least from the models in nature that we could compare it to—is one comprised of fruits and shoots, shoots being young tender greens. I believe there is a place for those young tender greens. They add a mineral density that we don't tend to find in high abundance in fruits. I believe the concept of fruitariansm has a good base. There are paleontologists and other research scientists who are looking into why we experienced hyperencephalization, which is a dramatic growth in the size of the human brain as compared to the other primates. It is theorized that brain growth and hence an increase in intelligence was due to the consumption of a readily available supply of high calories. Most of the current researchers are guessing that this meant consumption of meat, but they are carnivores themselves, so that is their frame of reference. They just guessed that because meat has a high caloric supply because of its fat content, we must have started eating meat to supplement our eating of leaves. Yet the discovery of nuts would certainly satisfy the requirements of the paleontologists who are looking for a calorically dense food supply. So would the consumption of fruits. Both are consumed by our

closest genetic cousins in the anthropoid apes and other primates. On a completely separate note, however, there are
other scientists who study animals. Most of them would be
considered field biologists. They have come up with their
own theories of intelligence. What they are suggesting is that
amongst all primates, there is a very interesting dietary prefer-
ence being discovered. Throughout the monkey kingdom, as
monkeys increase in intelligence, their fruit consumption also
increases. Amongst the anthropoid primates, those that are
our furthest genetic cousins—the least intelligent anthropoid
primates—consume a diet of almost exclusively vegetable
matter. The anthropoid primates that are our closest cousins,
the bonobo or the pygmy chimpanzee, who are the most intelligent of all the anthropoid primates, eat a diet almost exclusively made up of fruit, including only a little bit of greens.

Juicing

I'm of the opinion that whole fresh, raw plant foods, ripe
and organically grown, eaten as a mono meal or in simple and
acceptable digestible combinations, are the healthiest foods
that we can consume. Neither adding fiber to our food or removing the fiber from our food benefits us in terms of improved health value. If a person wishes to have a glass of juice
because they enjoy it now and then, I certainly wouldn't hold
that against them. I wouldn't tell them that they are never
going to go to "Hygiene Heaven" because of it. However, I
would say that they are doing it because they like the food
and not for its increased health or nutritional value. I think the
health value comes in eating food in its whole natural state
and that removing the fiber depletes the food in a wide variety of ways.

Sprouts

When I walk through the woods, a field, or wherever I
have gone walking in nature, I very rarely find sprouts. I think

many sprouts taste good. If someone goes through the effort of growing sprouts for me, I will eat them. I certainly will not shun them, but I don't in any way think that they are magical foods or special foods, better than all other foods. I would classify them as shoots, which make up part of our regular diet. In the rainforest I have occasionally found a seedpod that has fallen to the ground. In one little area you might be able to find 50 or a 100 sprouts that are coming up out of the ground that may or may not be edible. We never know for sure until we try them. So even if you find sprouts in the wild, you are talking about a little patch of 50 sprouts. Trying to make a diet of sprouts would be difficult in the wild, as you hardly ever find more than a few. I prefer and recommend foods that have a nutritional makeup that closely mimics our nutritional requirements. Most of these foods are fruits.

Natural Hygiene

Hygiene is the science of human health. I am all in favor of applying hygiene in my lifestyle and of teaching others how to incorporate the use of hygiene into their lifestyle. I believe that this makes absolutely the most sense environmentally and every other way that we could possibly evaluate it. Natural hygiene is a redundancy, I mean, what would "unnatural hygiene" be? The American Natural Hygiene Society as an organization, has suffered from the same quirks and the drawbacks as any other bureaucratic organization which has as its primary goal is its own growth. As a natural living activist and as a hygienic person, I feel that natural hygiene has helped a tremendous number of people to take a step along the path. There are many steps along the path and I applaud everyone taking steps. It is my belief that there are more steps to take beyond those taught by today's natural hygienists.

Supplements

For people who eat well and follow the other 32 tenets of

healthful living, supplements are in and of themselves unnecessary. For people who do not eat well, supplements will not make up for this lack of eating well, just as coffee will not make up for lack of sleep. Or an artificial tan will not make up for sunlight required to produce our own vitamin D and hence experience a proper calcium metabolism. There are times when anyone can get into a nutritional problem either due to aspects of their lifestyle or situations beyond their control, where a brief period of supplementation may be in fact life-saving. It's my practice to never sacrifice a patient's or a client's health for my own philosophy. I am not yet ready to die for my philosophy. If the only food around is cooked food and it's the only food that's going to be around for a long time, I will be tempted and probably will eat cooked food for sustenance, while I live on my nutritional reserves. I know that I have a good nutritional reserve and it will get me through that period. As an example, this interview is taking place in New York City, and although I strictly and only believe that we are pure air breathers, I'm not going to hold my breath for 4 days until I get out of the city. I believe that my life requirements supercede my philosophical ones. I do not think that supplements as a rule help anyone. Nutritionists estimate that more then 2/3 of all the nutrients on the planet have yet to be discovered. They know that all nutrients work in a coordinated fashion with at least 8 to 10 others. The simple math of this indicates that anytime we take a supplement, we are definitely creating imbalances with at least 5 to 10 other nutritional factors, and then in turn, 25 to 100 more.

Food combining on a 100 % raw-food diet. Do you think it necessary?

I think that the more correctly you eat, the more sensitive the human organism becomes to proper food combining principles and practices, and the more necessary food combining becomes. However, once again, my guidance for people is that food combining is a transitionary step toward more healthful eating. There are no animals in nature that provide us with a model to think that we are supposed to combine our foods. Even those animals that eat a wide variety of foods eat them one at a time. A bear eats berries and fish but he does not bring berries over to the fish and put berries on his fish. I think that food combining is a step along the way. It is one that people should know about. It would be wise if everyone made the transition to food combining. They could still eat all the foods they love, just in different orders. It is like learning to speak French instead of English. The verb comes in a different place. But, the place where we are really trying to guide people is towards eating mono meals of whole, fresh, ripe, raw, organic plants.

Exercise

I am not particularly fond of exercise. I am particularly unfond of the concept of workout. We go to work and nobody is particularly happy about it. We work on our relationships and it starts to have a negative connotation. I think work is a four letter word that ends in k and most of those are words that we don't use. I am not fond of the concept of work at all. If work was all that good, the rich wouldn't have left it to the poor. People work their whole life in order to retire so that they no longer have to work anymore. However, I am in fact very much in favor of an active lifestyle. I myself do not like to do anything indoors that I can do outdoors, nor do I recommend it. I have never been a proponent of weightlifting. However, I am a strong supporter of strength activities and fun strength-building games. Whether those are sports requirements, recreational activities that require strength, strength games, or whether this is just the use of calisthenic activities where we use our own body and our surroundings as the resistance. To me, going to the gym, indoors, to lift weights and put them back down, provides very little in the way of a meaningful activity. However, in terms of just pure strength activity it's hard to argue with the fact that people will build strength in the gym. I am not saying don't go to the gym if you really like it. I just would rather see people go climb a hill. Speed, strength, endurance and all other facets of fitness must be reinforced, or they will diminish. It is much easier to maintain fitness than to regain it.

Fasting, Water fasting vs. Juice Fasting

Fasting has two definitions. The first is "to hold fast." This originated as a nautical term, and refers to making a knot hold fast so that it stays put. When we do this type of a fast, we pick a food and eat that food to the exclusion of all others. This could be, for example, a water fast, a fruit fast or a juice fast. However, the second definition of fasting is in more common use today, and that is "to abstain from." In this case, when people do a water fast, technically what they would be doing is abstaining from water, although we use it to mean the exact opposite. When we say that we are on a water fast, we mean that we consume nothing but water. I think that there's very good scientific evidence to support water fasting or abstaining from all foods other than water when we do not feel like our normal selves. When we are extremely tired, hurt, or not feeling well, the best thing is to fast and rest until we are better. The beauty of the fasting state is that during this time all neurologic activities vector toward normal. Homeostasis is regained. The body more quickly resumes its vitality and recovers health while in the fasting state than in any other. Please understand that hygienic fasting refers to a state of deep rest. This includes all four types of rest. Physiological rest is induced through the reduction of eating. Sensory rest is achieved by going into a pleasant natural setting where the sounds that we hear are the soothing ones of nature. Emotional rest can only be found where we are in a supportive environment with people to take care of us. Physical rest is where all physical activity either ceases or is reduced to as great a degree as possible. True and effective hygienic fasting requires that we participate in all four types of rest simultaneously and drink only pure water.

What is your age height and weight, and talk about how your weight has changed through this diet, and how you have handled it?

You know, my age has changed through this whole diet too. I am currently 46 years of age. I can stretch myself up to five foot ten. I weigh approximately 150 to 155 pounds. I believe that is fairly close to my natural weight. In my adult life, I have reached a high of 180 pounds during the sedentary lifestyle of chiropractic college that was imposed upon me there. I was still a grain-eater at the beginning of chiropractic college. My lowest adult weight, after a month of fasting, was 100 pounds. I had no difficulty regaining muscle mass at all. On a Standard American Diet, my weight was normally 165. I always felt that it was too high. My body fat level varied between 10 to 15 percent on that regimen. Currently I maintain a body fat level between 4 to 5 percent, which I enjoy immensely.

Do you currently eat 100% raw foods and if so how long have you been eating 100% raw foods? Also, do you ever have any slip-ups and eat cooked food?

I've been a 100% raw foodist for 18 years and during that time I have experimented with the consumption of some starchy foods and with the consumption of some cooked vegetables on occasion. Most of those occasions have been the exception; for instance, the once or twice a year that I find myself at an event where suitable raw foods simply are not available. However, at one point during this period, I did experiment with a couple of months of near daily starch consumption. I think probably it was because my memory was poor and I forgot why I went off starch consumption in the first place. I would be the last person to tell you that cooked food does not taste good and that any of the foods that I ever ate in my life didn't taste good. I do not think that is the sole requirement for healthful eating. The food that I eat now certainly tastes good as well. In fact, most people have two requirements for food before the meal, but only one after the meal. The two requirements before the meal are: does it taste good and is there enough? But, after the meal the only requirement is: was it enough? At this point in my life, I do not tend to have slip-ups as far as maintaining my raw regime. I just spent a week at the European Vegetarian Conference. There was very little raw food and a wide variety of gourmet vegetarian food. I remained 100% raw. The week before that was the North American Vegetarian Society Summerfest and the same thing occurred. They made it very challenging to become or stay a raw foodist in the face of all that gourmet vegetarian food. However, I remained as a 100% raw foodist. I do not feel that I am missing out. In fact, I think that everyone else is missing out on high levels of health, vitality, well-being, good feelings and all the positives that come with the raw-food diet. I do not feel I'm missing anything. I think that it is the other way around.

What is your average daily diet like?

I maintain a fairly high level of activities. I train world-class athletes and very often workout with them. In fact, I just spent a week working out with the Austrian gymnastic team. They do some pretty serious workouts. I also workout with pro basketball players. There are three factors that affect our fitness levels: frequency, intensity, and time. I tend to participate in all three of those to a pretty high degree. Hence, I eat more than a typical person would who lives a more sedentary lifestyle. When I'm in a sedentary lifestyle, I eat only two meals per day. When I'm active, most of the time 3 meals a day supplies me with plenty of calories to meet my needs. Generally, my morning meal tends to be a juicy fruit of some type. It could be coconut water, melons, mangos, nectarines or something of this sort. This morning I had grapes. My lunch meal depends on the type of activities I have done that day. Some days I want more water, and others, more sugar. I will have either watery fruit or something a little more dense like bananas. Almost everyday, except during mango season, I eat bananas for lunch. I have friends that grow 75 varieties, so I have a pretty good choice of bananas. I usually start dinner with some sort of acid fruit, and follow that with a few or more of the following: lettuce, celery, tomatoes, nuts, seeds or avocados. I do know just from keeping track that I consume about 3500 calories a day.

What is your favorite food?

I have a top ten list of foods, and they are all fruits. The fruits on my top ten list most people have not heard of because they grow in the tropics. Certainly Rolinea, Iliama, Inga, Water Apple, Maranon, Mango, Banana, Mamey, Lychee, and Granadilla make the list. I haven't tried many fruits that I do not like. I usually feel that the best fruit I've ever had is the one I am eating at the moment. Without question, my favorite vegetable is celery, with lettuce taking a very close second place.

Of all of the fruits, do you think one is the most important?

No, I really do not think that there is a most important fruit unless you are extremely active. I think bananas or some other high caloric density fresh fruit, such as canistel, sapote, mango, mamey or lychee would have to take a primary role. Bananas really are the one out of all of those that are available all-year round, so bananas have to be one of the preferred foods for humankind, especially for extremely physically active people.

How's your health and energy level? How much sleep do you get, and think the average person needs?

My health is excellent. It's improving all of the time. My fitness levels I would say are excellent, but I am striving to improve them all the time and they are improving. My criteria for determining how much sleep to get is...did I get enough? I need enough sleep. I need to stay in bed until I do not feel like staying in bed anymore. But, in terms of hours of sleep per day, this typically requires me to sleep about 6 hours in order to feel that I've had enough sleep. However, when I increase my training or when I am trying to make strides in my training, I need more sleep than that. Eight hours is not uncommon, and ten is not unusual if I am really pushing myself physically. I put sleep and rest in a category together. When things are going the way I like them to go, I attempt to get 12 hours rest a day. Six or so of sleep and another 6 or so of rest.

OK, those are *your* personal sleep requirements, but is there an average amount for most people, or does it vary depending on their lifestyle?

I think it is different. It is unique for each individual. But I would say that six hours tends to be fairly common, and between 25 to 50% more sleep being required by the same person if they were consuming cooked foods only once per day. Maybe another 20 to 25% more sleep if they are consuming cooked foods 2 or more times per day. They could easily need 50% or more sleep, which would bring them up to 9 or 10 hours as a requirement for how much sleep they need.

What changes have you noticed mentally on this diet?

My memory has improved and my vocabulary has improved. My ability to think on my feet is much improved. My ability to stay on an even keel is unparalleled. I have no flare-ups in temper anymore, ever. Not that I had many before, but I did occasionally have them when I was on a grain-based diet. I am a much happier person. My outlook is more positive. I expect health and my health keeps improving. I think that I am more positive, happy and if I could say, more aware. I feel that my intellect is at a sharp edge on a raw-food regimen, and if I include cooked foods, it instantly dulls my mind.

Is there anything else you would like to add?

I'd like to recommend to people who are looking into the raw food way to consider it strongly. It is difficult to imagine what it is like to be on a raw-food diet from the outside looking in. I would recommend that they make the transition comfortably yet as rapidly as possible. A simple strategy for this might include something like one raw meal a day for a month and then 2 raw meals a day for a month. Then as time goes on 3 raw meals a day for a month as an experiment. If you like the results continue the experiment. If you are not happy with the result you can always go back. The cooked food will still be available, for sure. I think that people also need to realize the environmental impact of eating cooked food. The amount of fuel consumed in the cooking and cleaning that could be saved on the raw-food diet is astronomical. I am sure it mimics automobile fuel consumption. The positive impact that we can have on our planet is profound. We also know that the raw-food eater utilizes just 25% of the land required for a vegetarian whose diet includes grains. The vegetarian uses significantly less land to produce his or her food than does someone eating the Standard American diet. We could feed 40 times as many people on a grain based diet than we can on the Standard American Diet. We could feed 100 times as many people on a raw-food diet as we can on the Standard American diet. This would allow us to feed a lot more people and use a lot less land to do it. I encourage people to make the transition step by step. I urge people to seriously pursue this philosophy in order to achieve optimum health. The results are just fantastic, and I will continue to do everything I can to support people in this worthwhile and rewarding endeavor.

Dr. Fred Bisci

Fred Bisci is one of the nicest and most knowledgeable people I have ever met. He is kind and gentle. His knowledge about the human body surpasses most people alive today.

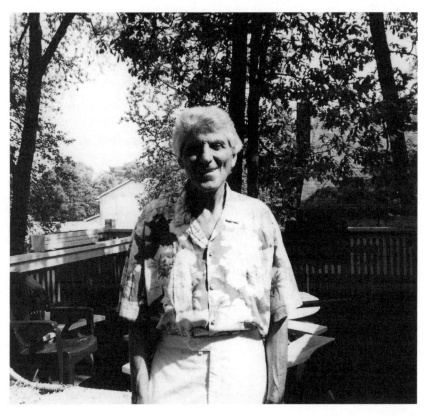

Dr. Fred Bisci at his home in Staten Island, New York

How many years have you been on the raw food diet and what got you into it?

I was always interested in nutrition. When I was a young kid, I was an athlete. I was also learning disabled. Little by little, I changed my diet. I would say about 30 years ago, I ran into a

267

fellow who was into eating raw foods. At the time, I thought he really was extreme or radical, but I always had an open mind. I have always been the type of person who did not settle for mediocrity. I always believed in striving for the highest ideals. Therefore, I decided to make a change and pursue it. The more I did it, I got to a point where I decided that there is no doubt about it, eating a raw-food diet is definitely the way to go. Since then, it has served me well.

How was your health when you started the diet?

Fortunately, I was always a healthy guy. When I started the diet, I was big and strong. I had very big muscles. I was into weightlifting at that time and was a good athlete. I came from an athletic family, so I never really had any health problems. I was not the type of person who got into this diet because I was sick. Illness is the main reason why many people first start eating the raw-food diet. However, I never had any major illnesses before getting into this.

Who have been some people who have inspired you to do this the most when you started out and is there one person that inspired you more than anybody?

I would not say there was one person that inspired me the most. Many influences impressed me greatly such the writings of Herbert Shelton. I had read just about everything on nutrition, and there was so many contradictory views out there, but Herbert Shelton's writings were very profound. They were very close to what science was saying and what you would learn in college about biochemistry and things like that. However, he just took it from a different approach and made you see that it was workable. I was always the type of person that made up my own mind, and I was always determined to find the answers out for myself. I was very careful and everything I went through I did systematically.

What do you feel are the most important factors in

eating a raw food diet successfully?

Not to be impatient and to persevere through it all. Understand that you are not going to get it down right away. You have to realize that the body releases endogenous materials, and you are going to have cravings. You are also going to have setbacks. It is important not to be discouraged. It is also important not to set unrealistic goals for yourself.

What are some pitfalls people getting on the raw food diet should avoid?

I think one of the major pitfalls is the negative feedback you are going to be getting from people around you, from your family and your friends who are not into it. I think you have to surround yourself with people that are knowledgeable and are into raw foods that have been successful at it. They have gone through it and have dealt with it very well. That will help you a lot. In addition, other pitfalls are the social ramifications, because if you are eating just raw foods, you are socially opposite to the average person. You will also have to be very careful about getting medical interventions once your body is clean as your body will be more sensitive and you might react negatively to pharmacologically-oriented medical treatment. In addition, I think most people have to go through a transition where they struggle a little bit and have cravings. I have heard of cases where people just go from eating a horrible diet to an all raw diet and do it successfully. I heard of it, whether it is true I do not know. I think it is a lot easier to go through the cravings and do it systematically. People also have to understand that they will go through periods of self-doubt. I know that's what happened to me. Therefore, those are some big pitfalls to avoid.

What are some common pitfalls people experience with weight-loss and teeth problems?

I will talk about weight loss first. There is a direct correlation between your diet and tissue quality. When you go to an all-raw diet, the average person's tissue quality is not good. The average American actually is like a walking pus bag. So you have to understand that when you make the change to an all-raw diet, your weight is going to go way down. When I first changed my diet, everybody thought I was making a tremendous mistake because I lost so much weight. I went from being a very well built guy to being like a toothpick. To do this successfully, you have to understand what is going on with the body. When I first got into this and went to some of the natural hygiene meetings, some of these people looked horrible. They were terrible examples of good health was. The reason was they were the people that were into the early stages of this diet. Their bodies were detoxifying and weight-loss was part of that. The people that were doing well were not going to the meetings because they already have been past that. Many people never get through this stage because there is so much confusing information out there that is misleading. Many people then and today, do not realize that the person trying the perfect diet does not always have the perfect body and because of this, they suffer in making the transition.

Now I will talk about teeth. Blood gases are connected to teeth problems. You have to be very careful, for if. your teeth start to become pain-sensitive, that means your stomach has a backpressure of gases. Your teeth are the first place you will feel pain if you have backed-up gas inside your blood. If this happens, the gases back up into your blood and that is where the trouble begins. It could also demineralize your bones in the roots of your teeth.

What do you suggest is the best thing to use for fillings for your teeth instead of mercury ?

There are non-metallic composite materials now available such as IPS empress and all the other new space-aged materials that are fantastic. There are several different materials you can use in place of mercury fillings. New porcelain ceramic is very good. I have some of those in my mouth. I have not had any problems with them. I find them to work well. I do not find them auto-intoxicating or poisonous in any way. I am able to tolerate them but everybody has to find out for themselves.

I am going to mention some topics. Tell me your opinion on them.

Nuts & Seeds

Some people have a problem digesting them. If that is the case, you should soak them. People have to find out what's best for them. Most people that seem to do well, do eat nuts and seeds. I know people that do not eat them, but you do not want to hurt yourself by limiting too many foods from your diet. You need a variety of different foods. I think people should try eating nuts and seeds. Make sure you soak them. Exercise beneficially speeds up your metabolism, and you will be able to tolerate the nuts and seeds much better because your digestive system will work much better.

Grains

I think in some respect, grains are worse than animal protein. If you are in transition and you have to eat grains, then you can eat them. If you want to you can sprout them to make them more digestible. Many people eat grains and have no problems. I have people that come to me who eat grains and overcame disease. It depends upon where you want to go and what your goals are. If you are aiming for an all-raw diet, you will get to the point where you cannot eat grains. It will just cause you to have mucus, joint pain and all kinds of problems. If you are not eating an all-raw diet, you can eat grains and be a healthy person, but once you eat an all-raw diet, it is not easy to go back to eating grains. You are just going to suffer too much.

Is the fruitarian diet sufficient in itself, or are some greens necessary?

Yeah, absolutely. Having greens in your diet is much safer. I do not recommend anybody to eat a diet of only fruit. I think that if you do that you will run into disaster. I have seen some people actually just about destroy themselves. People say they eat a fruitarian diet of only fruits. I do not have proof, but I think a lot of them are just telling tales.

Sprouts

If you are going to eat grains the best way is to sprout them. Are sprouts necessary? I do not think so. Part of the reason why many people on the original Hippocrates diet were so skinny is because they were eating too many sprouts and grains. They were getting too many endogeneous enzymes in their diet. That made it hard for them to put on weight.

The Natural Hygiene diet concepts

I think natural hygiene has validity, yet natural hygienists are certainly making mistakes. They might be overeating on fruit which raises the level of their blood gases. We have to look at the reasons behind what is going on today in Natural Hygiene, why so many natural hygienists are getting cancer. Many hygienists today are dying of cancer. One reason is they are not eating a sufficient variety of foods, eating too little green leafy vegetables. They do not understand the connection of eating fruit to their present bodily state. As time goes on, you can eat more fruit, however, if your stomach starts to extend, you start to get a gas-filled stomach and your teeth start to hurt, this means higher blood gases and fermentation. If that happens, you might be eating too much fruit. That means you should be eating more fats, more nuts, and eating a variety of different foods.

Supplements

They do not work the way people think they work. What they are doing is actually preventing the release of endogenous material. Many people start taking supplements, and they feel better. This is because the supplements actually prevent their body from detoxifying. I tell the majority of people who have come to me not to take supplements. For some people eating a mediocre diet, eating some chicken, fish and turkey, they may benefit from taking supplements. They are not going to harm themselves, but if your going into a raw diet, you should not take supplements. If you're going to eat a diet that's above 75% raw, supplements will end up making you sick some place down the road.

Hybridized Foods

I think many people are over-exaggerating the harmful effects of eating hybridized foods. I think you could have them in moderation and they will not hurt you. If you are eating any kind of cooked food, you can certainly eat hybrid food. You will not have any problems with them. If you are eating an all-raw food diet and you are never deviating, you will get to the point where certain hybrid fruits and vegetables might give you some phlegm. Just do everything in moderation, and you should not have a problem with it.

Eating Seasonally

Eating seasonally definitely has validity. I know a guy who is a natural hygienist that lives in Alaska. He was having watermelon flown up to Alaska and he was freezing to death. If you are living in a cold climate, you must have more caloric density from heavier foods in order to generate sufficient basal metabolism. You are going to have to eat some dried fruit, some nuts or some other fatty foods. Otherwise you are going to freeze. As time goes on and you become more efficient and cleaned out, you can eat that type of a diet. Then your body will be warm even in cold weather. However, not everybody is that way. If you are very clean inside and you are eating just fruits and vegetables when it is 20 degrees above zero out-

273

side, your body will generate enough heat. But if you are cold, you have to look at your diet. When you are cold, your body is contracting. You can take warm baths to help the blood circulate. This will warm you right up.

Fasting, Water Fasting vs. Juice Fasting

You have to understand what you are doing when you are fasting. Many people fast when they are in a crisis, but you have to understand that fasting is a crisis-creating situation in itself. In other words, if you are feeling well and you fast, then you will not feel good. You created a healing crisis. If you are already in a severe crisis and you are already weak, it might not be a wise idea to do a water fast, unless you are ready to go to bed, not move and keep your eyes closed. Another mistake that people make with fasting in natural hygiene is they are not drinking enough water. You actually should be drinking more water when you fast. The water is a transit medium. You need it to carry the endogenous waste out of your system. Many natural hygienists say drink water only when thirsty. I think that is a mistake. You should be drinking at least a glass of water every hour. Otherwise, you are going to feel terrible. Water fasting is more effective than juice fasting, but there is more risk to water fasting. Anybody that tells you there is no risk to water fasting and that the body will never harm itself, doesn't know what they're talking about. I know people who have died on a water fast. Now with juice fasting, I think it is very good. It is much safer and you will not get as weak. You can go about your business. If you have to function, you could function easier on juice fasting. Now, it is all relative as to how much juice. If you have three glasses of juice a day, that is enough to carry most anybody through anything. I know some clinics that give people up to 13 glasses of juice a day. That is really too much. They're really detoxifying and auto-intoxicating people at the same time! Many people are doing that and they do not even know it.

What is your opinion of the different lengths of fasts?

Unless you have a lot of experience with fasting, I would say you could fast up to seven days. Understand that breaking the fast is the risky part. I have personally seen people break a fast the wrong way and go into renal shock where they had to go to the hospital. I do not think there is anything wrong with fasting one day a week. I know some hygienists say that it is worthless, that fasting one day a week does not do anything for the body. I do not agree with them on that. I think fasting one day a week is fine. I think when you fast one day a week, what you are doing is you are giving your digestive system a rest. It might not be a therapeutic fast, because your body does not get into therapeutic fasting on a one-day fast. You are just cleaning up your system. I do not see anything wrong with doing a seven day fast once a year, unless you have a medical condition, if you have a thyroid condition or you are a diabetic. However, for a healthy person fasting seven days or doing a fast occasionally is fine. I personally fast often. I am a fasting person.

So you think it is healthier to plan a fast ahead of time than to fast when your body is asking for it?

That is correct. I think it is a good idea to plan a fast ahead of time so you do not get into a situation where you have to do it. Actually, the best time to fast is when you really feel good. As crazy as that might sound, I have done that many times and it takes you to a whole other level. However, when you do that you cannot go back. Once you're eating a diet that is an uncompromising type of diet, you cannot go back to a diet that is compromising. You always have to upgrade your diet.

Is food combining on a 100% raw-food diet necessary?

I think that you have to look at that on an individual basis. I know some people that are on raw diets and they do better when they combine their foods correctly. I know other people on raw diets that do not have to combine their foods. I could just about mix up anything, but I notice a difference. I am not saying I will not suffer for it, but everything relates to energy. You are going to have to expend more energy if you are mixing your foods up. If you do not mind combining foods, I think it is a good idea. If you are already in transition and you are in true biological healing, I recommend that you do combine your foods. If you do, you will heal much sooner, and you will not feel as bad. I tell everybody that comes to see me to food combine. As time goes on, I call them to see how they are doing. Then they can start to deviate a little bit. If they could tolerate it without having many problems with their stomach, then and only then is it OK not combining your food.

Wild Foods

Wild foods are excellent if you have access to them, but only if the food is whole and there are no chemicals on it. It must grow naturally and it have its full complement of nutrients. It must be fresh and eaten right away.

Sea Vegetables

I think they are very important. They are a great source of nutrients. They are high in sodium. Your body can handle that kind of sodium. I tell people to incorporate it into their diet. I eat seaweed myself. Dulse and kelp are my favorites.

Exercise

Fantastic, if you are eating a good diet and you are very healthy, you should have such an abundance of vitality and energy that you want to go out and exercise. If you are eating a raw diet and you do not have a very strong desire to use your body, that means there is something wrong and you are making some mistake. You have to use your body, just as a wild animal uses their body. They are constantly roaming. They do not have to exercise. They are always fit and able. If you are eating a raw diet, you are automatically fit. A person that's eating a raw diet, if they wanted to go out and run they should be able to run 5 miles very easily without any trouble and without any training. So yes, I think that exercise is very important. Anything that involves movement I believe is very good for you.

What is your age, height and weight?

I will be 70 next year. I am 5'11. Now I am about 10 pounds lighter than I normally am. So my normal body weight is usually between I would say 140 and 150. Right now, I am about 138 pounds. Normally I am heavier. I could gain weight easily if I want to. I eat a very small amount of food. For me, the basic premise for eating is not to gain weight.

Would you talk about your weight change and other changes your body has gone through on this diet?

Years ago, when I first started I was an Olympic weightlifter. I weighed well over 200 pounds. I had a very solid physique. When I got into raw foods, everybody thought I was crazy because I lost so much weight. I got down to a very light weight. One time I went on a long water fast and my body weight was down to 100 pounds or even less. Whenever you are going to a raw-food diet, even if you are already thin, your body weight is going to drop. It is a frightening experience for many people. I have seen a woman go down to 70 pounds. You are going to get a lot of static from people. The feelings are very scary. You have to be careful.

Did you ever go through a bad detox?

Yes, I did. When I was a young guy, I ate a lot of animal protein. Whenever you are a weightlifter and eat a lot of protein, the detox is extremely difficult for that type of person. That is why my detox was so hard on my body. I had a guy come to me recently. His wife was sick. He was a big guy and he worked out with weights. He said, "I will eat this way with her and it will not bother me." He lasted two weeks. He went into detox and he couldn't take it. He was scared to do it and it was too hard on his body for him to do it.

Do you currently eat a 100% raw food diet? If so, how long have you been doing this for? Do you ever have slip-ups?

Let me explain the whole story. When I first got into a raw-food diet, I was going back and forth. I would go a month or two, and then I would slip up. I would have tremendous cravings. They were very hard to control at that time. I would skip eating for a couple of days. Then I would get back into it. I went back and forth there for a while. Then for about 12 years, I ate all raw. Then I went through a period where a couple of my brothers died. I was discouraged, so I started eating some steamed vegetables again. When I started eating steamed vegetables, right away it opened up the gate for cravings, and I saw that I was going to slip into oblivion again and start eating starches. So I knew that wasn't for me. Therefore, I went back into eating a raw food diet. Now, very rarely will I eat anything that is cooked. Maybe I might have some steamed vegetables but I have not done that in years. I will not say I will never do it again. I am not paranoid about all this. However, I know if I eat anything cooked, I get ill or I fall right to sleep. Therefore, my diet is now strictly 100% raw.

What is your daily diet like? What do you eat and how often?

I very rarely eat more than twice a day. Most of the time it is once a day. Today, all I had was two papayas, a banana and an avocado, that is all I ate, and I am not planning to eat anymore. Tomorrow morning I will get up and I will juice. I like juicing. I also like blended salads. I eat a lot of them. I like to use cucumbers or coconut water as a base. Then I throw in romaine lettuce, spinach, and I might throw in some dandelions in it.

Then I throw in some flaxseed oil, or maybe some raw flax seeds, some avocado and a little bit of kelp. I whip it up and make a delicious blended salad, and I have a nice big bowl of that.

What is your opinion of the practice of juicing?

I think the natural hygienist are wrong in thinking that you shouldn't juice and that eating the whole food all the time is always better. I lived on juices for a long time, and I was fine. The only thing is that it's another step up. You have to be ready to do that. If you do that, you have to be careful because if you go back to eating some of the other things that you were eating before, you will not tolerate it as well. I do not see anything wrong with juicing.

You have mentioned that fruit is your favorite food. Of all the fruits, which is your favorite?

I really like watermelon and mangos, but my favorite food by far is figs, I love figs.

When it comes to food, do you feel it is important to eat every single food grown organically, or are there some inorganic foods you can get away with eating?

Well, it depends upon whether the chemicals penetrate below the outer layer of the fruit. I think avocados are probably OK. Sometimes I eat them even if they are not organic. You are much better off eating everything as much as you can organic. The added chemicals mimic estrogen in the male and female body. They lower the male sperm count and they elevate the female estrogen levels. That is why there are so many estrogen-related cancers. What's going on today with all the chemicals they are putting in food is a disaster. I think that eating organic is very important, so make sure you do the best you can.

Of all the foods, do you think that there is one food

that is more important to eat than any other food?

Not really. I think the key is to eat a variety of foods. Make sure you are getting a variety of different classes and categories of foods. The need for protein is over-exaggerated. We are obsessed with protein in this country. If you are getting enough calories, unless you are doing something radical, most likely you are getting enough protein. I think the basis of diet should be fruits and vegetables.

Currently how is your health and energy?

My health and energy is fantastic! I will be 70 next year and I have the same vitality of when I was 35, maybe even more so. I only sleep 2 to 3 hours a night. I have been married for about 25 years and my wife has never seen me sick, so I would say my health is very good.

How many hours of sleep do you think a person should get every night?

It depends on the condition of your blood. When you are sleeping your blood is dialyzing. If your diet is terrible, you might need 12 hours of sleep. If you are going through biological healing, you need as much sleep as you can get. You might need 15 hours of sleep. However, as I said, it all comes down to the condition of your blood. The cleaner it is, the less sleep you will need.

What changes have you noticed mentally on the raw diet?

It is astounding! When I was very young and eating cooked food, I was always in trouble in school. I was also learning disabled, and I had a speech impediment. Now I am fine. Here is how you have to look at it. Man only uses 8 to 12 percent of his brain. Where is the rest of his brain? It all depends on the condition of your blood. That is the result of your diet. When you get into an all-raw diet your blood gets cleaner. Many people go to the Middle East. They start chanting and meditating to develop elevated consciousness. All you have to do is go on a good diet and clean up your blood. Then your mind starts to work better. Then your consciousness will naturally become elevated. Diet is the key. I cannot stress it enough. Your mental equipoise and the sharpness of your mind all depends on the condition of your blood, which, in turn, is based on your diet. You can change unbelievably.

In your opinion, are eyeglasses and contact lenses necessary?

I wear glasses. There was once a period that I wanted to get rid of them. I tried to give up my glasses with the Bates method and I saw that it was working, but I did not go through the whole process. I feel anyone could do it naturally, without drugs or lasers. If you have to continue to wear glasses, so be it. I know plenty of people that have given them up by doing eye exercises. There are glasses out now with little holes in them that strengthen the eye muscles. Yes, it is possible, but I have not done it. Therefore, I can only speak for myself in this area.

Not many people talk about the blood gases. Where did you learn about it and could you tell us what you know about it?

Arnold Ehert wrote a little about the gases but I did not learn about it from him. I did a lot of long-term fasting, and I learned about it from my own experiences. There was a gentleman in Brooklyn though, he was probably the most knowledgeable person on this planet about this and nobody has ever heard of him. Somebody told me about him and said he was a maniac, that he was a nut. They told me what he said. I thougth, wait a minute, this guy is not a nut, he knows more than anyone else does. I spoke to him a few times about blood gases. He said he would not teach me but he gave me some clues. He told me that once I understood it, I would find my way from there. He was right about the gases. I picked it up, and I found my way from there. I think that the blood gases are the most important aspect of health. Most people have no clue what is going on. If you learn to understand the blood gases, you then understand why we develop all these diseases, even if one eats raw foods.

Is there any more information you can give about the blood gases?

What happens is that when you overeat on fruits and mis-combine them, they stay in your stomach and ferment inside you. Once that happens, the gases backup into your blood, and that is where the trouble begins. Here's how it works: The body is composed of trillions of cells. Each cell is like a mini-factory. The waste products from the cells are gases. When you are eating, the body is accommodating exogenous material which means you absorb food into your system. Then as you start to eat better, your body starts to release endogenous material. The endogenous material consists of solid waste and accumulated toxins. That is when you start to get into the gasses. The gasses cannot go from a low-pressure to a high-pressure area. Therefore, if you have flatulence, you may have h-pylori bacteria. You are eating too much fruit, and you have a bloated stomach. The waste gases will not come out when this happens. You give some off when you exhale, but it will not go into the alimentary canal and cause you to pass the gas. That becomes a back-pressure, the waste endogenous gasses, which are supposed to permeate tissues, come into your bowels, and you pass them out with your fecal material. Your body can become like a sponge full of water. That is what the gas is. If that happens, then the gasses backup into your blood and that is where the trouble begins.

What degrees do you have?

I have a Ph.D in nutritional science.

Is there anything else that you would like to add?

I would just like to say that a big problem today with diet is people are starting from the wrong premise. They are starting from the premise that you have to eat animal protein to be healthy, that you have to eat dairy products to get enough calcium. This is why people can never come to the right conclusion. It is like dealing in mathematics. If you try to solve a mathematical equation and you're starting with the concept that one and one is eleven, you will never come up with the correct solution. That is what people are doing today and did traditionally. They thought you had to eat that type of a diet to be healthy—like eating chicken, fish, and turkey—and that eating anything outside of that diet could not possibly be healthy. They also thought that about having dairy products, eating plenty of bread and cooking your vegetables to death. So that's what is a large part of the problem.

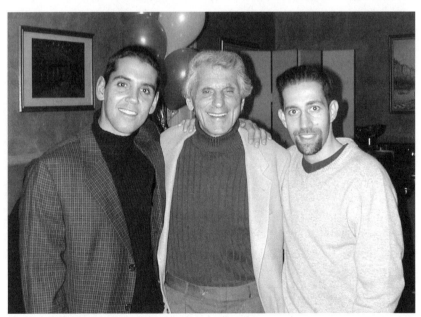

(left to right) Enrique Candioti , Fred Bisci and Paul Nison - Oct.2000

Roe Gallo

Roe Gallo is a great woman. She has more energy than anyone I know. I never met anyone who is as happy as her. She is always smiling and happy. She contributes her energy and happiness to the RAW LIFE.

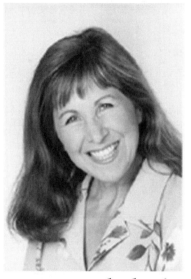

How long have you been on the raw food diet and what got you into it?

In 1975 I began a dramatic change in my eating habits. I was on steroids due to an asthmatic condition, which was getting progressively worse. After a water fast and lots of research, I discovered that the best food for our physiology is fruit.

Who have been some people who have inspired you to do the "raw life" and is there one person who has inspired you more than anybody else?

No one in the beginning. What inspired me initially was a strong desire to live.

What are a few of the most important things you have learned in order to do this diet successfully?

Keep it simple, eat to live, then go out and have fun.

Are there any pitfalls that you have learned to watch out for on the raw food diet?

The pitfalls I have seen are overeating and eating too many concentrated foods such as dried fruits, nuts, etc.

Common pitfalls people come across are with weight-loss and problems with their teeth. Could you comment on those issues?

Most people store excess fat in their bodies. Even thin people usually store fat and not much muscle. So losing the fat may make a person look "too thin." Rebuilding the body with muscle is a slower process, so patience is important.

The people I know who have experienced problems with their teeth are the ones who do not practice good oral hygiene. Cleaning the food out of our teeth by brushing and flossing is essential.

I am going to mention some topics. Tell me your opinion on them.

Nuts and Seeds

They are concentrated and hard to digest.

Grains

They are concentrated and hard to digest.

Is fruitarian diet sufficient, or are greens necessary?

Fruitarian diet is complete, yes. Some greens if you like.

Sprouts

No!

The Natural Hygiene Diet concepts pointing towards a 100% raw food diet?

Absolutely, cooked food is very difficult to digest.

Supplements

No! You have to digest supplements. Why bother doing that to your body.

Eating Seasonally

Yes!

What about fasting? Would you recommend water fasting or juice fasting?

Fasting yes. Juice fast: a citrus juice "fast" most people can do until toxins are almost completely gone. Water fast: a water fast most people can do for a day or two without supervision.

Do you think it is necessary to fast only when your body is asking for it, or is it ok to plan a fast?

Fasting is great to clean out toxins. For those who are without symptoms, planning a fast would be fine.

Exercise

Absolutely, it is important to nourish the muscles.

Wild Foods

If you find something that is not poisonous and tastes good to you, then eat them.

Sea vegetables

Yuck!

What is your opinion of the female cycle concerning the raw diet? Do you think it is natural and healthy for a woman to stop bleeding during their monthly cycle?

Usually there is some flow but if you are healthy, it is light and easy. I stopped bleeding 2 years ago. Last year, I did a blood test that told me I was postmenopausal. I never had a symptom.

Is it natural for a woman if she completely stops menstrual bleeding, to have a light discharge?

It seems to be. My period used to be very light and sometimes only a slight discharge. It is hard to say for sure because there are not enough healthy women to track patterns.

What is your age, height and weight? Could you talk a little about how your weight has changed from when you first went on this diet?

I was born 12-17-49, so I am 50 this year. I am 5'3 and weigh about 102 pounds. My weight changed and I have gotten much leaner.

When you first got into this, did you lose a massive amount of weight?

I lost about 20 pounds.

Since starting the raw diet did you ever get sick or have a bad detox?

I started with a water fast and yes, I was detoxing from steroids. It was intense.

What percentage of raw foods do you eat now and how long have you been eating this way? Do you currently eat 100% raw foods?

Yes, now I am eating 100% raw fruit, mostly organic. I used to go back and forth from eating 100% fruit to eating mostly fruit (90-95%) with a little fun food thrown in (sometimes the fun food was cooked or processed). But even with 90% fruit, the 10% fun food started to make me feel tired and sick. Who needs that? Now, back on an all fruit diet, I feel fabulous. In 1975 I started eating 50% fruit, but by 1985 I was up to 90% plus.

What is your average daily diet like?

What I eat changes with the season. The quantity depends on how much physical exercise I am doing. I like to keep my weight at 102 so I eat enough to keep me there which comes out to approximately 2-6 pieces of fruit per day plus 2 to 3 quarts of water or orange juice and water together.

Out of all of the foods, do you think there is one that is most important?

Yes, I feel fruit is the most important.

What is your favorite food?

Ripe sweet fruits.

How is your health and energy?

My health and energy are great.

How much sleep do you get and what do you think is necessary?

I generally get between 5 and 7 hours of sleep. The amount of sleep you need will depend on your overall health, on how much energy you use during the day. A good rule of thumb is to fall asleep when you are tired and wake up without an alarm.

What changes have you noticed mentally on this diet?

I started this when I was very sick, so I could see a dramatic change in my mental health.

Is there anything that you want to add before we end it?

Thank you... Remember the body (mind, body and spirit) is one unit. Take care of the whole package. Be kind, loving and joyful. Think good thoughts, do good deeds. Eat fruit, have tons of fun and smile.

Brian Clement

Brian introduced me to the raw-food lifestyle. I met him in Florida years ago, and I am so glad I did. He was my stepping stone in the transition from a cooked life to THE RAW LIFE. He is very knowledgeable about the lifestyle and through his health clinic, The Hippocrates Health Institute. (HHI) I would say that Brian has changed more people's lives in this movement than anyone else out there today.

How many years have you been acquainted the raw food diet and what got you into it?

It's been 30 years. I went into it naturally after being a vegetarian for about 5 years before that. The difference between the vegetarian diet and the living foods diet was so significant that I remained this way.

How was your health when you started the diet?

It was fair to medium. Being an average vegetarian, I was eating too many carbohydrates and never feeling the energy level that I should have. This was because I was not getting oxygen from the food and all the other elements. Once I got on the living foods, after several months, I started to recognize probably a doubling in my strength and in my energy.

Who are some of the people who have inspired you towards the Raw Life? Has there been any one person that inspired you the most?

Many people have inspired me, but the person who has inspired me the most is Dr. Christine Nolfi. Dr. Nolfi actually coined the term, "living food" some 75 years ago, after healing herself of breast cancer. After her, some other people who have inspired me were Ann Wigmore and Viktoras Kulvinskas.

What do you feel is the most important thing you have learned to be successful at eating a raw food diet?

One thing we recommend strongly here at Hippocrates is that people consume a wide variety of fresh sprouts. The reason being is because nutritionally they are much more nutritious than vegetables or fruits. The second thing that we have learned is that the consumption of juices made with green vegetables and sprouts are significant for healing. What I have learned personally from this is to be humble and do not take it too seriously. Live your life and have fun. Also, understand other people and their reactions towards you, towards what you are doing. Remember that at one time it was not easy for you either.

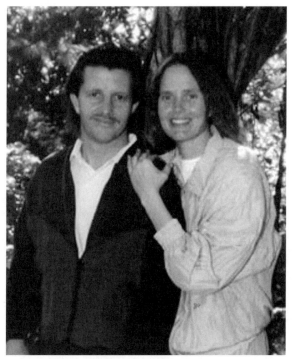

Brian with his wife Anna Maria

What are some pitfalls that you have learned to watch out for on this diet?

That people tend to want to eat too many sugars and that is because we are all addicted to sugar from our former lifestyle. It is a common thing for people to want to eat a lot of dried fruit and sweet fruits. It is also a common thing for people to want to eat a lot of bread, even if it's sprouted and not cooked. You should avoid a lot of that. The only people that should be eating large amounts of sprouts and sprouted grain items are people who are athletic and doing muscle training exercises.

I am going to mention some topics. Tell me your opinion on them.

Nuts & Seeds

Certainly they are good, but in limited amounts because they slow the bloodstream, and they can create problems with the gallbladder and liver. You should always soak nuts and seeds before eating them.

Grains

I recommend that in the sprouted form anyone can eat them, but the amount that one needs is basically the amount of effort and exercise that that person is doing. We put athletes on a whole lot of grains and non-athletes on minimal amounts. Sprouted grains are the best way to eat grains. There are many different kinds of grains. Some are better than others. I would say Millet and Quinoa are two of the best.

Is the Fruitarian diet advisable, or are some greens necessary?

Greens are very necessary in the diet. You must make sure you get a lot of chlorophyll into your diet. Eating greens and drinking green juices will make sure you do that. If you do not eat or drink greens, you will run into some serious problems.

291

I highly recommend everyone get some greens into their diet everyday. As for the fruitarian diet, I believe that fruit today has way too much sugar, and we should not eat most fruits. Here at The Hippocrates Health Institute, only a very small percent of the diet consists of fruit. I think it was a viable diet when we began as the human race. Without question, humans definitely ate that way. When the fruit was ripe, it would fall to the ground and you would eat it and spit out the pits. What happened though, at least what we know from the writings that are at least five and a half thousand years ago, the fruits were hybridized. They mixed them together. They did this to decrease perishabilty. They had to grow them in colder climates and hybridization made them more resistant to the colder weather. Hybridization made the fruits much sweeter and when it first happened that is what the people took into account. From what we know, the average fruit today has thirty times more sugar than the original. These high amounts of sugar no longer make them a truly natural food. We also have to take into consideration that we pick most fruit today when it is not ripe. When you consider these facts, you could almost be sure that they are mineral deficient.

Sprouts

They are simply the best food you can eat.

Supplements

Most supplements are not whole food supplements and are not good. They are made of chemicals and are a waste. However, the use of whole food supplements will help when somebody is ill. It will also help someone who is healthy and an athlete. When I talk about whole food supplements, I am talking about living food supplements. I only recommend whole food supplements. Supplements are important in helping people at HHI get their bodies back to the health they desire.

Eating seasonally

A good concept back in time, but not today. This is because nowadays, people are always moving around. It is not easy to eat foods in season. It does not mean much today because foods do not grow in their true location. I think it is more important that people eat food that is organic and as fresh as they can get it. Most important, make sure the fruit you do eat is fully ripe.

Fasting—Juice Fasting vs. Water Fasting

Well, we no longer think water fasting is viable for the body. I think juice fasting is excellent. Not on fruit juices, but on green juices. I fast one day a week. I have been doing that for almost three decades now. I highly recommend juice fasting over water fasting because water fasting puts too much stress on the body. Your body needs the benefits of the vitamins, minerals and enzymes of the juices. In addition, many people who come to Hippocrates Health Institute are diseased, and their bodies could not survive on a water fast.

Is food combining necessary on a 100% raw food diet?

Yes, I think it is necessary to follow the rules of food combining. There is no question about it. Anybody who does not agree with that is incorrect. It is especially true if you are on a 100% raw diet because the foods have all their enzymes and it will throw you off even more if you do not follow the rules. I hear many people say if you are 100% raw, you do not need to follow food combining rules. I think that is not grounded in biochemistry.

Exercise

It is very important. Especially if you want to put on weight. I think all exercises are good and important, but I would say the two best without a doubt are rebounding and swimming.

Wild Foods

If they are truly wild that is great. Many of the foods that people are calling wild are not truly wild. I think you have to be educated and learn how to find wild foods and identify them. If you could do that, then I do think it is great.

The Natural Hygiene Diet

It was a good, basic diet; unfortunately, there are some problems with it. Many helpful raw food practices we do today comes from the Natural Hygiene movement years ago. It helped us all get where we are. God bless it!

Problems with teeth when on the raw diet

It is simple. Too much sugar will cause you to have problems with your teeth. Fruits today have too much sugar for us to be consuming. This is because all fruits are hybrids. That is why many people eating many fruits have teeth problems. This is especially true for citrus fruits. In addition, another thing that causes teeth problems is eating fruits that are not truly ripe.

Problems with weight-loss

We have to realize that food, especially if it is raw, will not put weight on our bodies. You cannot put any extra weight or be fat on a raw food diet. Natural foods will not let that happen to your body. That is why to put on weight people must incorporate strenuous physical exercise (such as weightlifting, Hatha yoga, etc.) into their life.

What is your opinion of colonics?

I am a believer that in the early stages of health transistion that colonics speeds healing for people. I would never do a colonic or an enema without following it up with an implant. To help the intestines heal, I recommend taking an implant of wheatgrass or algae after colonics or enemas. They are great.

What is your age, height and weight, and would you please talk about how your weight has changed over the years. In addition, talk about any other changes your body has gone through.

That is an excellent question. I am about 170 pounds. I am in my 50's. I am 5'9. When I started this program, or this way of eating, back when I was 24, my weight was 240. I was very sick. As I said before, several doctors told me I was dying. The asthma I had was killing me literally! I had a hard time walking up stairs. When I went on the program of living foods, my weight dropped all the way to 119lbs. The physical strenuous exercise that I did helped me redevelop my body the way that it needed to be developed. The best food for one's body is living food. When you switch to a living food diet, you will get very thin. It is not an optional thing. If you do not exercise, you will stay thin. Anybody at any age can put on good weight by doing exercise and sticking to the living-foods program.

Do you currently eat a 100% raw food diet?

No, my diet is 80% raw foods and 20% cooked. The cooked food being good organic vegan foods. Many days during the week I do eat 100% raw.

Knowing how bad cooked food is, is there a reason you do not eat 100% raw foods?

I would say there are social reasons. I think it is important to be able to relax and eat with family, friends, and not have to worry about if the food is all raw. Physically, there is no question that 100% raw food is best.

What does your average diet consist of and how often do you eat?

I eat two meals a day consisting of big salads with an avocado, some grains and always sprouts. I have green drinks everyday, several times throughout the day. Juiced sprouts, mostly sunflower sprouts are in my green drinks. Wheatgrass juice is also something I try to drink everyday.

Would you say most people eating a raw-food diet as long as you have been, are still eating a 100% raw foods?

I would say probably the majority are doing what I am doing. Because in the beginning, you have to be very strong. Whatever it takes, do it. After you do it a long time and attain a good level of health, then you loosen up a little bit as long as you do not go too far backwards and let it get to you mentally and physically.

Is there one food that you think is most important?

I have done tests and concluded that sprouts and salt water vegetables, sea vegetables, are the most important. They are the best choice out of all the foods. Buckwheat and sunflower sprouts are the best sprouts. Wheatgrass juice is also very important.

When it comes to doing the raw diet in a cold climate, is it harder to do because of the cold weather? Is it physical or more mental?

Absolutely a mental thing, and I will prove it to you. Every food must be absorbed at body temperature. When you eat cold food in a warm climate, like ice cream, your body has to heat it up from below 32 degrees to 98 degrees. If you are in a cold climate and you eat a hot food let's say it is 125 degrees, your body is going to have to cool it down to eat it. Now there is some physiology involved here, but the bottom line is to take food and heat it up, or to cool it to bring the temperature down, both take the energy out of your system. To do so you will make yourself colder physically when taking in hot food than you will to make yourself warm.

How much sleep do you get? What do you think is the average amount of sleep a person should get?

It is different for everyone. I am a person who has a very

stressful job dealing with sick and diseased people all day here at HHI. I need about seven to eight hours a night because of that. When I was younger and ate fast food, I used to sleep much more. I remember traveling the world with Ann Wigmore. She could get by on three or four hours and be up with a lot of energy all day. Therefore, it depends on the person and their lifestyle. I think the average amount for the average person is eight to eight and a half-hours a night. There are exceptions but that is average. The majority of people I know that switch to a raw diet, the amount they sleep is dramatically reduced. If you are on a raw-food diet for some time, you could get by on five or six hours and do very well.

What are some changes you have noticed mentally on the raw diet?

What happens is that once a person's biochemistry starts to function well, the brain starts to work better and more oxygen will flow to the brain. The effects are a feeling of euphoria, a sense of feeling good and calm. With that, it allows an individual to become a better person and thus allows us to be doing what we should be doing. When you are on this diet, the way you look at everyone changes, and it just takes everything to another level. It is a great feeling.

What is your opinion about interpersonal relationships when making the change to a raw diet?

It is hard to be with someone who is not supportive. As I said, being humble and compassionate is so important. When you eat natural living foods, you become more humble and compassionate, so it should not be hard for many people to get along with others. When you eat more raw foods you should and, I hope you do, understand and feel for other people. It is not easy for people to change their diets just as it was not easy for you at one time. It is important to understand your lover's feelings. However, I hope people have the guts and they are brave enough that, if they are not happy in their relationship or in their life, to make the necessary changes they need for them to become happy. Even if that means leaving your partner.

When one makes the transition to a raw food diet, do you find they think about sex more often or less?

I would say the whole experience becomes clearer. After a person goes through the initial detoxification, the ability to have sex becomes more defined. When a person is being unnaturally stimulated and eating many non-foods, they will trigger an abnormal desire for sex. Therefore, they are like rabbits running around. When the raw foods cleans out their body, they will not desire it as often. When they do, it will be more meaningful and their endurance will be much better. This is because once the raw foods clean out their body, they are stronger and healthier. In addition, more oxygen will flow to their sexual organs. Because of this oxygen flow and the hormone balance, the whole experience is changed.

What is your opinion on the positive effect of raw diet on the menstrual cycle? Do you feel it is natural and healthy for a woman to stop bleeding when on a raw food diet?

In the majority of cases I have seen, I would say, yes. However, diets that people are on in the living-food movement or raw food movement lack fatty acids. If that is the case, then they are not eating a wide enough cross section of foods. That might cause the bleeding to stop and it is not natural. However, in most cases it is a very natural process. I know that there is a primitive tribe where the women have blood during their cycle only twice a year. An odorless gel comes out the other ten months of the year. It is not just from the raw-food diet. They are just anatomically stronger than us. If you stick long enough to a living-foods diet, you generally get rid of PMS along with the pain and the suffering. All of the women on the Hippocrates Health Institute program have noticed their menstruation has become dramatically less.

Is there anything you would like to add?

I would just like to add that I think the more people get involved with the living food lifestyle, the better people are going to be and the better humanity is going to be.

Morris Krok

Morris Krok's writings are the best there is. Morris has by far written more great books than anyone has about the raw-food movement. Book after book he says it all in just the right words. His books have changed my life. I would have to say he is the greatest living raw food author. He is still thriving and looking great. Meeting Morris was one of the greatest days of my life. My only regret was that it wasn't long enough. The information Morris has is invaluable. No money could ever buy what Morris has taught so many others and myself. He is my idol. I look forward to his future writings and one day spending more time with him.

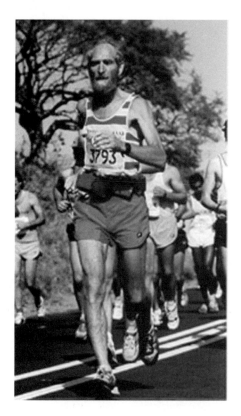

Why is it important to internally cleanse the body before eating food?

Is Ehret right in saying that we should break a fast with a fairly large amount of raw food, especially a salad and not high sugary fruits?

Why is adequate rest important?

How much food should we eat on a daily basis?

Why is it important to be strict when on the raw diet?

If a person is having problems with digestion and elimination on the raw diet, what should he do?

When is the best time to eat?

What is the raw diet's biggest pitfall?

What is the problem of eating too many concentrated raw foods?

What is the most important things you have learned over the years?

What is the true cause of ill-health?

What is the best healthy way to live?

What is the secret of youthfulness?

What is your opinion of exercise?

Any final thoughts?

ANSWER

Let me see if I can do the impossible by giving one answer to the following questions that you put to me. In my attempt to reply to all of these questions, my intention is to explain what method really works and why we do not need to know very much in order to achieve a higher state of health, as the key is to follow some simple basic rules.

Many of the above questions overlap so the answer in my opinion will be found in understanding how our body functions and what are our basic needs. Two important concepts will also be brought to your attention.

One deals with the phenomena of withdrawal symptoms and the other is following Tony Officer's wise injunction to cleanse the system internally.

Our physiological structure indicates we should eat those raw foods that we find palatable. It can be fruit as well as tender and pleasant tasting leaves, flowers and roots. If we were brought up on such a diet from birth we would not have any digestive troubles as the system would be in such a clean state with no organs impaired that the overeating of some of the more concentrated raw foods would not be a serious problem.

The raw food principle contends that when eating raw food the body will assimilate what it needs and eliminate easily, without depleting nervous energy, which is superfluous to our needs. Foods that can cause problems are the high sugary foods such as dates and dried fruits. Too much high sugary foods because of being so concentrated are acid-forming and an indication that we are eating too much of it is when brown wax builds up in the ears.

To overcome this problem dried fruits should be soaked or eaten with things like carrots or greens. Dates should also be eaten in this manner. Nuts if eaten in excess are acid-forming, and some of them, even though they contain oils, can have a dry consistency. Almonds in particular, our most alkaline nut, falls into this category. Here again, nuts are best eaten with carrots or some tender leaves, and they are certainly more palatable with raisins. This latter combination is not recommended by natural hygienists who contend that the best form of eating is to eat only one type of food at a time; and that the fats in the nuts do not go well with the sugars in raisins. Both nuts and dried foods eaten in excess can produce thirst.

The best way to eat grains is to sprout them and in most cases to eat only the sprout. Raw milled grains because of their high starch content can result in mucous accumulating in the digestive tract. The body has not the mechanism to handle starches raw or cooked very well. Too much raw grains can also produce thirst. It should be obvious that the best raw foods are those that are organically grown and unsprayed. Oils such as olive, linseed and the other vegetable oils should be used sparingly as they can be heavy on the liver and clog up the lymphatic system. They are best used as a salad dressing mixed with some lemon or cider vinegar. Taken this way the oil is diluted and it is broken up into smaller particles that will ensure that it is easier to digest.

The most harmful foods are the starches, especially those that have been refined, dairy products and animal fats. All these substances disintegrate in the warmth of the digestive tract into sludge, although they appear to have food value and keep hunger at bay. They in fact transform the body into a dirty drain, and in time will cause all our illnesses from a cold to the stiffening of our joints and muscles. We are as young as we are supple.

As raw foods are digested with greater ease, they result in the body unloading all the harmful substances that has been soaked up into the tissues since infancy, including the saturation of slime that has accumulated throughout the membranous tract from the anus to the sinuses. Withdrawal symptoms is based on the physiological law that the moment we cease eating a toxic forming food, that toxin is released into the general circulation for elimination. As this can be unpleasant, imbibing once again that harmful substances, will seem to be the cure as it will suppress that symptom. It is for this reason that toxins have an addictive effect.

To obtain the best results from changing over to raw foods, is to internally cleanse the system by living on water and diluted fruit or vegetable juices for at least five days and where possible even longer. It is only fluids that can dilute toxic substances in the body and help wash out the thick slimy substances that have accumulated. In the beginning one should not have less than one glass of fluid every two hours. After a few days one can increase the amount of fluid drunk. This quantity of water will help to cleanse the stomach walls and small intestines of some of the slime that has accumulated in the digestive tract overnight. We may find slime is also passing out of the colon on its own or with the stools. But because man has accumulated so much over a lifetime, the body cannot be cleansed in a few days.

Tony Officer, an original health thinker who intuitively conceived his morning cleansing system and explained in his book, *Why Grow Old* said one of the most profound health statements that I have ever read. He wrote, "Anything that remains behind in the digestive tract the following morning is best washed out." If one follows this rule, it certainly becomes the best way to start the day.

It may not be necessary to eat a large amount of food when breaking a fast. Five or more glasses of water could achieve the same peristaltic effect. As the fast has rested the digestive the tract from a great deal of work, even a small amount of food can result in some bowel evacuation, if of course, there is still faeces present. When the body is very efficient, one can experience a bowel movement after every meal.

According to yoga, three months are needed provided we are ultra-strict to purify the system. Even when we have ceased living only on fluids, there is no harm drinking a few glasses of light water that has been allowed to stand in the sun in between meals, first thing in the morning or 45 minutes before eating, even if there is no thirst present. By including water in this manner, we will prevent sweet fruits from becoming sickly. My experience is that five or more glasses on an empty stomach has a refreshing effect on the brain and results in the spontaneous release of enlightened thoughts . Many of my sayings have come as a result of this practice.

When the body is fairly clean, even the eating of one apple can keep us satisfied for a few hours, and if we include some of the more concentrated foods, we may feel very satisfied on just one meal for the day. Raw foods as their fibrous structure is intact and they have not been transformed by heat are more sustaining than cooked substances.

The benefits that are derived from fasting (it is only a form of cleansing) and raw foods will prove that there is no such thing as a specific illness, nor are there are specific remedies. It will also indicate that it is not true that we must daily eat so much protein, fats, carbohydrates and calories. Good health is based more on a balanced health style than on taking supplements, vitamins and minerals to overcome a so-called deficiency. The real illness causing factor is a system clogged with unwanted substances. Internal purity is the way to keep the body young and supple.

When the body has been thoroughly purified, then the processes of assimilation and elimination will begin to work with clocklike efficiency; and in fact operate simultaneously, becoming one operation. Also, as the body and mind is one, and consciousness is present in our every cell, health of the body will present us with the most wonderful gift of all—a mind replete with clear resplendent thoughts. The yogis referred to the awakened mind as the thousand petalled lotus.

Morning sickness shows how the body attempts to keep

the female organism as pure as possible to achieve a healthy pregnancy and birth. As nausea and biliousness are the most unpleasant symptoms that we can experience, to mitigate them, drink on awakening, five or more glasses of warm water. This will make it easier for the body to vomit effete matter that has collected in the stomach and intestinal tract overnight. Yogis from ancient days and also some primitive tribes have used this method to purify the digestive tract. This method is so helpful that it can be referred to as Health's Magic Wand.

The common cold is the first indication that our body is becoming saturated with toxins, slime and other unusable material. It is not primarily caused by germs. It must not be suppressed with drugs or other unrelated methods, but allowed to run its course by simply living on plenty fluids until such time the entire membranous tract is clean. What causes a cold will eventually cause practically every other symptom. A more severe form of a cold is influenza, or a fever of one kind or another. When you understand what a cold entails, there should be no mystery why we become ill.

Immediate benefits are obtained from what can be referred to as the "no-substance elements." We will be energized and refreshed, even if it is only in a small way, the moment we breathe deeper, expose the naked body to fresh air and the sun rays, and gently stretch every muscle and joint in the body as Hatha Yoga advises. These yoga postures will be beneficial even if done in as little as fifteen minutes a day. They can be repeated a few times a day if one so desires.

To be healthy we do not need to have big muscles to run marathons, or swim the English Channel, or even do yoga exercises. Normal activity during the course of the day should be sufficient to maintain optimum blood and nervous circulation. All the no-substance elements including a shower, a cold water sponge, or just walking barefoot on the dew, will have an immediate beneficial effect. It is not like the eating of food where the benefit is only found hours afterwards when it has been completely digested, and the body and mind have been freed from this activity.

The benefit we derive from eating or from exercise can only come about by the rest interval between these activities. The mind, also, functions better when we give adequate time to absorb and mull long enough over any new teaching or piece of information. It is less efficient if it is cluttered with too much in too short a time. Zen and yoga teach the necessity of emptying the mind through meditation so that its surface can be so polished that it once again can shine and reflect inspired and original thought.

Life is nothing more than moments of consciousness, but for these moments to be meaningful, do not interfere with the intelligence within, as only when it is unimpeded that it can do its work efficiently. Also, the voice within will speak more eloquently when we cease impressing it with theories, beliefs, preconceived ideas, and rituals that have no link with reality. When the mind is calm and the breath is silent only then can we become attuned to universal wisdom. The most intelligent thing we can ever do is to put ourselves in the gears of elimination. It is only in this mode that those substances hindering the finer workings of the body will be removed.

Several of Morris Krok's great sayings:

*"More murders are enacted in the
kitchen than anywhere else."*

*"In ten minutes you can eat so badly
that you will become an invalid for a week."*

*"Cleanse the stomach so that the purified
mind can be forever inspired."*

*"Nothing is more detrimental to man's
advancement and well-being than an untruth
which is given authoritative approval."*

*"There is no truer saying than we are
what we eat, or to put it more strikingly
-what we eat eats us."*

*"Health cannot be stored, it must be
earned everyday of your life."*

I hope you have enjoyed these interviews as much as I have. Read them repeatedly. Each time you will pick up something new. Such valuable information. Learn it, live it, and have a great RAW LIFE!!

9 | RAW CURIOSITY

Common Question and Answers

I feel good eating cooked foods. Why is eating raw foods so important?

It is important to eat raw foods because they are perfect foods for the human body. If you keep putting the wrong gas into your car, after a while your car will not run as well as it should. The same thing will happen with your body if you continue to eat cooked and processed foods. Eating cooked foods were not intended by nature. We are supposed to eat our food raw and whole. If you think you feel good on cooked foods, wait until you eat a raw-food diet. Everything your body needs to survive—and live to its fullest—is found in raw fruits, vegetables, and nuts.

What is so bad about cooked or processed foods?

It is very unnatural to eat cooked or processed foods. Processed foods already have essential nutrients removed. And after cooking even whole foods, many important nutrients are destroyed, so then your food lacks the nutrients your body needs to thrive. Worse, many cooked foods clog up your body with thick, slimy waste. If you continue to eat them, you will not feel well. If you do not stop, you will suffer from toxemia, or even worse, you will die.

Is there any scientific evidence that the raw food diet is as good as you claim?

Dr. Doug Graham gives lectures all over the world about the raw-food diet and says, *"All sciences point to the consumption of raw food as best for the human body. The science of nutrition, that is establishment textbook nutrition, mentions raw fruits and vegetables as the best source of every known human nutrient. No organization is promoting cooked food for its nutritional value. Logic dictates that raw is best. There is no model in nature for the consumption of cooked foods."*

What is Toxemia?

Doctors have created thousands of different names for diseases of the body. However, there is only one true disease and it appears in different forms. This dis-ease of the body is called toxemia. Allowing too many harmful things to get into your body causes disease. Examples are cooked food, pollution, even negative thoughts.

Roe Gallo states it beautifully. Here is what she says about disease: *"Most conditions that we refer to as disease are preventable. Degenerative genetic conditions are not preventable, but they are also rare. Common conditions, such as cancer, diabetes, obesity, arthritis, asthma, allergies, heart disease, high blood pressure and atherosclerosis, although they are pervasive, are usually preventable. These conditions are not really the disease, but the symptoms of disease. The disease is toxicity. You create toxicity with poison and deprivation. The causes are poisoned air, water, food, thoughts (fear), and deprivation of nutrients, movement, rest, sunshine, oxygen and love."*

Is a raw-food diet too hard for people to follow in

today's society?

No, it is actually easier to follow than other diets. When you eat all your food raw, you do not have to waste time cooking or preparing your food. You just pick up your fruit and greens and you're ready to go. It saves more time to eat raw foods than eating cooked foods. Think about it, you always see people on the street walking and eating some sort of fruit, a banana or an apple, but you rarely see anyone walking down the street eating a hamburger or a steak. Also, it is much cheaper to eat raw foods and you can get them almost anywhere you go.

If I chose to eat some cooked foods, are some cooked foods better to eat than others?

Yes. If you must eat cooked foods, eating baked squash or lightly steamed vegetables is preferable to cooked grains, beans and other heavier foods. An alternative to eating cooked foods are dehydrated foods. Dehydrators make foods taste cooked, but the enzymes remain in the food, as long as the food is dehydrated at less than 110 degrees fahrenheit.

If I go on a raw diet, where will I get protein and vitamin B-12?

The body gets sufficient protein from the raw foods that you eat. You do not see wild animals counting protein grams. They get all they need from raw foods. You see how big and strong they are. All the protein and vitamins that your body needs, as well as vitamin B-12, are contained in raw foods.

In today's modern, unnatural diet, there is too much protein anyway. People have been brainwashed into thinking they need large amounts of protein to survive. It's just not true. In fact, excessive protein will cause toxemia in the body because it is unnatural for human beings to eat so much protein. A balanced raw diet contains the perfect protein concentration for our bodies.

The same goes for vitamin B-12. Our bodies only need very little B-12. If your body is clean of toxic waste, it will make and use its own vitamin B-12. If you want to get B-12 from raw foods, you can add sea vegetables to your diet.

I live in a cold climate. Do I need cooked foods to keep my body warm?

No! In fact, eating cooked foods in cold weather will make you feel colder. If it is cold outside and your warm body goes into that cold, you will feel colder. Why do you think that when you see people drinking hot liquids, they look so cold? Your body will handle the cold weather much better on a raw diet. This is something many people, including me, have noticed since switching to a 100% raw diet.

Is it important to eat seasonally?

Check out the interviews in this book. Those people interviewed said it best. It is not as important in today's modern, unnatural world to eat seasonally because we use air conditioning in the summer and heaters in the winter. But it is still preferable to eat food that is as close to natural as possible. If a pineapple grows in Hawaii, and you eat it in Hawaii, that is better than eating it far away in New York. The reason it is not as good in New York really has nothing to do with the weather. The pineapple just takes a longer time to get to New York, whereas in Hawaii, you could probably eat it as soon as it is picked. There is nothing wrong with eating a pineapple in New York in the middle of winter. It might be very cold outside, but inside your house, where you are eating, I am sure it is warm and cozy.

Is it hard to relate to others and adjust socially on this diet?

No, it is not at all hard. At first, people might think that your are weird. But that is because they are unnatural and do not as yet understand. The longer you are on a natural diet, the easier it will get for you socially. For many people, without even looking, they find a new group of friends who feel the same way they do about being natural. Actually, it is more likely that they will find you first. You will have such a good time with natural people who think the way you do that you will have very little time for unnatural people in your life. In time, your social life will be better than it was at the beginning of your dietary and lifestyle change.

Can anyone at any age eat this diet?

Yes, but although people refer to it as a diet, it is actually not a diet. It is a natural way of eating. Raw food is the natural food for every person and animal. The longer you have been eating unnatural foods, the harder it will be to make the change back to eating raw foods. But yes, raw foods is for everyone. *"You do not become natural; you were born that way."* You have been brainwashed; you have become unnatural. It is just a matter of getting back to nature and the natural diet. This is where you started from and where you should be, today and always.

Is there too much sugar in a natural diet of mostly fruits?

If you are eating what your body truly craves, the answer is no. There is much more unnatural sugar in today's modern, unnatural diet which people eat everyday. Once you are clean inside, your body will crave what it truly needs. Remember that anything with seeds is a fruit. Many non-sweet fruits will be included in your diet also. When you become natural, you will learn to love non-sweet fruits such as cucumbers, red peppers, zucchini squash and all others with seeds that might not taste good to you now.

Is it healthy to raise my child on a 100% raw-food diet?

Yes, it is not just healthy, but also highly recommended. This is how all babies should be brought up. I highly recommend that all pregnant women who are interested in raising their baby as nature intended read *Primal Mothering in A Modern World* by Hygeia Halfmoon. Too many people are poisoning their children with unnatural foods. You do not have to be one of them.

Sometimes you refer to a natural diet as consisting of raw fruits only. Are you saying that these are all I should eat?

Fruit should be the main part of your diet. I highly recommend you include these in your diet along with leafy green vegetables, seaweed and some nuts. They are all natural foods. When I refer to a natural diet, I am speaking about all of them. I have met with people all over the world who have eaten a raw-food diet for many years. They all feel that these foods are all that is needed for the body to thrive.

Is eating 100% raw foods boring? Are there many food choices that I can eat?

Eating 100% raw foods is definitely not boring. You could eat one fruit everyday for the rest of your life and still not taste all the fruits of the world. Do not limit your choices. Learn about and experiment with exotic fruits. There are many great tasting fruits that people do not know about. Learning about them will keep this way of eating very exciting.

I recently started eating a 100% raw-food diet, but I have had some problems, mainly loss of strength and loss of libido. Why is this?

Loss of libido is just part of the healing process. This does not happen to everyone on a raw diet, but do not worry. Stay on the raw diet and, in time, you will ignite your libido like never before. As for strength, when your body is detoxifying, you will have less strength. Go with the flow and rest during these times. When your body heals, you will be stronger than you were before you started eating raw foods. It is all part of the healing process, and it just takes time. Do not worry and have patience.

I thought a raw diet would give me much more energy, but I am eating 100% raw foods and I feel tired. Why is this?

There are times during detoxification that your body will need rest. At these times, you will have less energy than you are used to having. Do not fight it. Give your body the rest it is demanding. The longer you are on a raw-food diet, the less you will feel this energy drain. However, at the beginning, you might feel it more often. Detoxification takes a different amount of time for each person. In time, you will feel much more energy than ever before. However, if you overeat or do not follow correct food-combining rules, energy will drain from your body, regardless of whether or not you are eating a raw diet. Be careful about this.

How much water should I drink if I am on a raw diet? What is the best type of water to drink?

Drinking a great amount of water upon rising each day is the best way to start the day. It helps cleanse the body and wake you up. I suggest drinking 6 to 8 glasses of water upon arising every morning. The best type of water is the water found in organic fruits. The next best water available to most of us is distilled water. Be careful with water sold in plastic jugs, as the plastic will leach into the water. It is best to drink water that is kept in glass jars and that is at room temperature. Do the best you can.

What is your opinion about juicing?

I think juicing is excellent when you are in transition from cooked foods and other unnatural, processed foods. Juicing will help your body get all the natural, raw nutrition that it needs. When you are on a 100% raw-food diet, juicing is good if juices are all you can obtain; but eating the whole food is always best and most natural. Be careful not to overdo the juicing of sweet fruits and sweet vegetables such as carrots and beets. Try to limit your amounts, and dilute your juice with water to make it less concentrated.

Why do people have trouble putting on weight when they first start out on a 100% raw-food diet?

There could be many different reasons. In my opinion, I think the two most frequent are the following:

1. When people start eating more healthfully, their metabolism speeds up and their body burns more calories.

2. Your body is still dirty from unnatural foods. Until it is clean, your body will not be able to absorb nutrients from food, no matter how much you eat. This includes raw foods. The best thing to do is to clean out the body before starting a natural diet. This can be done by some sort of cleanse, a fast, and taking colonics. Once your body is clean, you should have no problem putting on weight. However, before starting a raw-food diet, you were most likely overweight anyway, so do not expect to get back to the same weight that you were on the unnatural diet.

Is fasting a good idea?

When your body is cleansing or going through a detoxification, fasting will help it get rid of waste much faster. Fasting on water, while abstaining from any form of food, is the only true fast. However, a juice diet can be just as helpful to the body as fasting on water. Sometimes it can even be safer and more beneficial.

If you decide to fast, never do so without the advice of knowledgeable people to help and advise you. Be careful how you break the fast too. For more information on fasting, read the interviews in this book. In addition, see the recommended reading section for many other good books on this subject.

What is a colonic, and what is your opinion on their value?

A colonic is a water flush cleanse of the lower intestines. A certified colonic therapist administers the process. A colonic involves slowly injecting water through a sterile tube into the intestines. When the water is released, stored up intestinal toxins and old feces are removed. The main purpose of a colonic is to aid the body in removing toxic waste that your body has difficulty removing on its own. One session is the equivalent of up to 15 enemas. Even though colonics are not natural, I recommend that at the start of a switch to a raw-food diet everyone get a series of 5 to 10 colonics to help clean out all the toxins and dirt that has accumulated in the body. The colonic therapist can advise you on how many you will need. After the initial colonic series, it is a good idea to get one or two per year (for maintenance) during the first two years on a natural diet. This advice applies only if you are eating a 100% raw-food diet. If you are not, then I suggest a colonic series at least twice a year, until you do switch to 100% raw foods.

What is your opinion about supplements?

I don't believe in vitamin supplements. If you eat a raw diet with a lot of variety, you will get all the vitamins you need. However, there are certain supplements you can take in addition to your diet. For example, enzymes, green powders and probiotics. These things can be very helpful. It is important to get a good quality brand if you do use these products.

What is your opinion about exercising?

I think people put too much time into planned exercise. My advice is just to do it. Anywhere you can get exercise, get it. Walk to the store instead of taking a car. Or take the steps instead of an escalator. You do not have to go to a gym to exercise. You could get exercise in your everyday activities. I think the best exercises for the body, and the most natural, are calisthenics. Walking and stretching are also excellent. You should try to do some exercise everyday. The main thing to focus on is movement. Make sure you move everyday. Walk everyday as much as possible. Mentally, meditation is "exercise for the mind" which I highly recommend.

I work out with weights. Could I maintain and increase my muscle buildup on a raw-food diet?

Engaging in any strengthening exercises will help you tremendously if you want to put on more muscle mass. When first switching to a raw-food diet, you might lose some muscle mass, but your muscles will grow back as long as you work them the correct way. In fact, they will grow much faster than they did before you ate a raw-food diet. You will get much stronger on a raw-food diet.

As an example of how strong you can get eating raw foods, look at the gorilla. A gorilla is the closest animal to man in terms of anatomy, and eats a 100% raw-food diet. Gorillas are one of the strongest animals on the earth. If gorillas ate any cooked food, they might get a little heftier, but they would not be nearly as strong as they are now. Two good books which I recommend for those interested in putting on muscle while eating a raw-food diet, are *Raw Power* by Steve Arlin of Nature's First Law and *Nutrition and Athletic Performance* by Dr. Doug Graham.

What is instinctive eating and what is your opinion of it?

Instinctive eating is based on eating what the body instinctively asks for through cravings. It consists of eating 100% raw food, including raw animals and raw fish. I know people who eat this way and have had some success with it, but I also know some who have almost died from it. I never met a person who has not had complete success on a 100% vegan raw-food diet.

I personally do not think it is natural for a human being to eat animals or fish, raw or cooked. I think that, except for encouraging the eating of animals, the diet has some good advice to offer. I believe however, that when we are not clean, our natural instincts do not accurately reflect our needs. All the abuse we have put our bodies through in the past has made them unnatural. Until we are clean, our instincts cannot be 100% accurate. If you eat animals, your body can never be clean enough to effectively engage in instinctive eating. For these reasons, I would be very wary of this diet.

What is your opinion of eating nuts?

It is very easy to eat too many nuts. As far as I know, no commercial nut on the market today is sold raw. They are all heated except when you get them from the tree yourself. You might still be able to find raw nuts at a local farmers market. Many nuts that remain on store shelves for prolonged periods also go rancid. However, they would do so even faster if they were raw. If you eat nuts, it is best to store them in a refrigerated place. Be sure to eat nuts sparingly if you decide to consume them.

10 | RAW TEST

Five questions to answer again

Now is the time to answer the same five questions that you answered at the beginning of the book. The answers are on page 322.

1. Who can keep your body as healthy as possible?

A. A Medical Doctor

B. A Holistic Doctor

C. A Specialist

D. Yourself

2. Cooked food is necessary to live a healthy life.

   A. True

   B. False

3. A vegetarian diet is deficient in protein.

   A. True

   B. False

4. The food you eat has no impact on your health.

   A. True

   B. False

5. For a happy and healthy life, a natural diet of raw fruits and vegetables is best.

   A. True

   B. False

Here are the answers to the five questions. If you did not get each one correct, then I suggest you reread this book. It is important to know the truth and the facts about your body and your life. Question anything in life that doesn't make sense to you. Just because many people believe something doesn't make it true.

1. **The answer is D.** Yourself. If you got this wrong the second time, please reread this book. It is important to know your body and nobody knows your body better than yourself. If you don't, no one will. Medical doctors do not study health, they study drug therapy. Don't listen to them. For good health, listen to what your body tells you.

2. **B-False.** If you got this correct the second time, congratulations! That is another fight you have won. If not, please reread this book.

3. **B-False.** If you got this correct the second time, congratulations! That is another fight you have won. If not, please reread this book.

4. **B-False.** If you got this correct the second time, congratulations! That is another fight you have won. If not, please reread this book.

5. **A-True.** If you got this correct the second time, congratulations! That is another fight you have won. If not, please reread this book.

If you've gotten all of these questions correct the second time you took the test, you are a champion and on your way to becoming a legend. Congratulations!

"So many people in this world are doing the wrong thing. When people start disagreeing with you, then you are most likely doing something correct. When they agree with you is the time to question yourself."

11 | RAW CONCLUSION

I have learned about health both from the experiences discussed in this book as well as from what I have seen and been through myself. I do not talk or preach to people whom I feel do not care to listen. When it comes to issues relating to being natural, I try to live by my motto *"Don't speak, just listen and answer only when asked."* I seem to be doing fine with that. This was my chance to say what I had to say, without having been asked. After all, the chance to express my views is one of the many reasons that I wrote this book.

I ride the subway everyday. As I look around at the people and their faces, what I observe is a shame. There have been days when I am the only person, in a full subway car, who is not sleeping. Most people have become very distant from nature. The reality is that many of them do know they are distant from nature, and even more sadly, will not do anything about it. The more natural I become, the more I notice how unnatural others live. I will not let this get to me. It can be very scary and disturbing to know the truth about people and about the world we live in. As much as I would like to make excuses or look away from the horrific facts, I realize that doing so will not change anything. The only way to make a change in what is going on in the world is to face the truth and stop looking the other way. Stop making excuses. If you want to change your life, this is exactly what you must do. *Face the truth!*

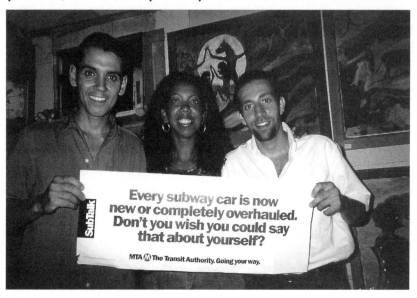

Enrique Candioti, Ana Vicenti and Paul Nison

This is an ad from the New York City transit system. If the biggest subway system in the world, which at one time was incredibly dirty, can clean up, why can't you?

I used to think there were just different types of people in the world who all thought the same. What I have learned is that all people are the same, they just think differently. There are some people who, when they are finished reading this book, will want to continue getting back to nature or as close to it as they possibly can. They will put their best effort forward to do so, no matter how challenging the task may seem. They will seek out more information and will continue to learn and grow.

Then there are the other people. They will say that making a change is too much work and not worth the effort. They will continue to make excuses for the rest of their unnatural lives. One of the most common excuses I hear from them is, "We are going to die anyway no matter what we do. Why should we bother making any changes." I think it is important to make the effort. Yes, you an I are going to die one day. But do you want to spend the last 20 to 30 years of your life in and out of hospitals, with sickness and disease? Or, do you want to spend all your time feeling the best that you can? Do you want to live your life like a true champion some of the time, or all the time?

Another excuse I often hear is "You could get hit by a car or have some other kind of accident and die tomorrow, so why worry about 30 years from now?" I tell them, "It is you who should stop worrying about dying tomorrow and start thinking more about living to your fullest. If you die tomorrow or 50 years from now, don't you want to live every second of your life feeling like a true champion?"

Then, there are the people who just don't understand. Sometimes something is very obvious, but people spend a great deal of time anyway, searching all around and looking for answers. The one place they forget to look is where the answer actually lies, right in front of them. I guess it is because, in most parts of the world today, most people have been brought up to look wherever they can to get the answers that they want to hear. Many people do not want to hear the truth, because it involves work, so they listen to the lies. Those are the lies with which you have been brainwashed. Now you have found the truth. Whether you want to use it depends on what kind of person you are. If you choose to get back to nature, the information is available. You now know where to start.

> *"Nature alone heals and only through complete acceptance of Nature's teachings can the survival of civilization be assured."*

—Arnold Ehret from *The Definite Cure of Chronic Constipation*

Face the truth. Starting this moment, only think pure and natural loving thoughts. Put those thoughts into action. Do your best to get all negativity out of your life and replace it with positive thinking. It all starts in the mind and in the way you think. Do not believe that you cannot make a change. You can and you will. No matter how natural you are now, continue to become more natural. Keep growing and never stop. Pray everyday. Spread peace, love, and joy to all; do unto others as you would have them do unto you. Have faith in a higher power, and you will live a happy life. No money is involved here.

You will be rewarded with a gift that is very valuable—that gift is good health, and it's free! Not just in the body, but also in the mind. Help others in life reach their dreams and you will be rewarded even more. Always remember the word "clean." Clean stands for **C**an **L**ove **E**nlighten **A**wake **N**ature. Your reward will be to have the best quality of life possible. The more people you help, the better quality of your own life. You will be happier and feel better about yourself. Don't hold resentment or hatred towards anyone. You want to live a life with no problems, so do not create any. Think of yourself as a crystal vase. Any unnatural or negative thoughts will create a scar on that vase. Make your life a spotless, shiny, clean, crystal vase. All the good things you put into that vase will always be with you. Live life with all those good things, and you will suddenly realize that you have become as natural as you can be. You have become a champion. Congratulations!

Life is great!

A raw life is a rawsome life!

A rawsome life is a great life!

Have a great raw life!

RAW DICTIONARY

People who eat a raw food diet often use the words and phrases below. This list will help you speak with them. There are different ways to eat the raw food diet. Each approach has its own philosophy. Be willing to experiment to find the one that works for you. Be original, but allow your belief system to serve, rather than imprison you. Life is change! Enjoy!

Anapsology: The philosophy and practice of Instinctive Eating.

Bioacidic Food: Of all foods, these are the most life-destroying and disruptive of vital force. All cooked flesh foods, processed foods, refined foods and foods with artificial additives and preservatives are bioacidic foods.

Biostatic Food: Foods that are not life-sustaining or life-generating but more slowly diminish the quality of body functioning, speed aging and encourage cellular degeneration. Examples are cooked foods or raw foods that are no longer fresh.

Bioactive Food: Foods capable of sustaining and enhancing existing vital force. Examples are live, uncooked unprocessed fresh fruits and vegetables.

Biogenic Food: Life-regenerating foods capable of dramatically increasing the body's vital force. These foods are rich in enzymes, predigested proteins, nucleic acids (RNA & DNA), and vitamins. Examples include tropical, high water content sweet fruits that are absolutely fresh and therefore a concentrated source of vibrant energy from the Sun; sprouted grains, legumes and seeds, cultured foods (nut yogurts & cheeses, fermented seed sauces and live raw sauerkraut.

Breatharian: The purified body of a fruitarian or vitarian has become so efficient that it seldom requires food & is mainly sustained by the energies present in sunshine, water & air. Breatharianism is said to be the last stage through which one passes before regaining physical immortality. If one were to progress beyond breatharianism, the body would be entirely transmuted into Light & that person would then be called a Heliovoran. Some have pretended to be breatharians, but there are others who seem genuine.

Jasmuheen is a woman who claims to be a breatharian and who actually teaches others a process she claims can enable others to become breatharians. True Breatharianism does not mean the body never requires food at all, but simply that through healthful living, the body has reached such a state of metabolic efficiency, that little food is required. When a breatharian is living in an environment that allows them adequate sunshine and fresh air, that person may require so little food that some people around them think they never eat. Contrary to previous theories, authentic breatharianism is never arrived at by forced dietary restriction. It is arrived at only by completely supplying all the true needs of the body once the body has reached a state of extreme metabolic efficiency,

Endogenous: From within the body—metabolic waste that accumulates when the body's vital force has been depleted.

Enervation: When nerve energy is depleted we are said to be enervated. Enervation leads to toxemia because nerve energy is necessary to remove body toxins.

Exogenous: From outside the body—from food or other substances we swallow, water we drink, air we breathe (also, anything absorbed through the skin including injections).

Fletcherize: To chew or masticate food very thoroughly. In the 1800's American Horace Fletcher popularized the notion that each mouthful of food should be chewed many times for maximize assimilation. Eating in this manner allows the body to heal many disease. It also allows one to thrive on a less quantities of food while remaining healthy. Adherents of the macrobiotic diet are advised to chew each bite up to 100 times or more. They must do this: for if they did not, they would be unable to extract adequate nutrition from their overly starchy grain-based diet. If raw food eaters did the same with the optimal diet of fruits, vegetables, nuts & seeds, the health benefits would be far greater.

Food Combining: Correctly combining foods to improve digestion. (Indigestion leads to enervation and toxemia.)

Fruitarian (or frugivore): A fruitarian lives only on fruit. Fruitarians are not limited to sweet fruits, but can eat any foods which contain within itself the seeds for its own propagation, Examples are: Squashes, tomatoes, cucumbers, avocados, etc. Some fruitarians also eat nuts, and justify their consumption by stating that botanically, nuts are a fruit which evolved without outer fleshy coverings. Natural Hygienists believe we are frugivores (juicy fruit-eaters), but that we also need some vegetables, nuts & seeds.

Heliovoran: This was our original condition at the beginning of creation when we required only God's Love & the energies of the Sun for our sustenance. We explored the universe at the speed of thought in "Bodies of Light." Our Bodies of Light remain, but garments of skin (earth, water & air) now veil them. It is said of Enoch, who conversed with angels: "and he was not, for God took him." Kaballah teaches that this means Enoch did not experience physical death—God directly "translated" his physical body into a body of fire in the process known as "Ascension." This body of fire of the ancient Hebrews corresponds to the Rainbow Body spoken of by the Buddhists. The Tibetan yogi Milarepa attained the *Rainbow Body* and could fly through the air.

Instinctive Eating: A philosophy of how to select and eat food according to instinct as do animals in nature. A person who eats instinctively may be called an "instincto" or an "anapsologist." Some instinctos eat only fruit, vegetables, nuts & seeds. Some actually eat raw meat. Most raw food eaters shun these folks! The truth is, you can eat instinctively without meat. Some instincto's claim otherwise, but that is really just an excuse for their nasty carnivorous habits. You can eat instinctively whether you are a natural hygienist, fruitarian, sproutarian, vitarian, liquidarian, or breatharian.

How to eat instinctively:

1 Select food exclusively from raw, organic, whole foods.

2 Select food instinctively by attractiveness and smell.

3 Eat that one most attractive food until it stops tasting good.

4 This taste change is your instinctive signal to stop eating that food.

5 If hunger persists, select another food.

Instincto-therapy: The use of Instinctive Eating as a thera-peutic modality. Instincto-therapy healing centers in France help people heal from a variety of diseases.

Liquidarian: Liquidarians do not eat solid foods. They take only fresh fruit & vegetable juices, coconut water, or pure water. Some liquidarians chew their fruits and vegetables, swallowing the juice & spitting out the pulp. Liquidarians obtain many of the benefits of fasting while continuing to consume their liquid foods. If your diet consists primarily of water-rich fruits, you will obtain many of the benefits of the liquidarian regime.

Mono Diet: Eating only ONE species of food at a time; which conserves vital force and takes less digestive energy.

Natural Hygiene: The philosophy and practice of eating pre-dominately raw fruit, with some vegetables, nuts and seeds. Natural hygienits feel this is the ideal diet for which nature has adapted us. They do not eat meat, dairy, grains, sugar, oils, condi-ments or spices. Nor do they not take vitamins, minerals, herbs or drugs. They occasionally fast for the purpose of rest and re-juvenation. They believe only the body "cures" & that all drugs are poisons. They try to procure pure air, water & food, ade-quate rest and sleep, sunshine, regular exercise & emotional balance.

Nerve Energy: A term used by Natural Hygienists meaning "Vital Force."

Raw Food Diet: This means the practice of:

1. Eating ALL of your foods RAW, or UNCOOKED.

   If you're not 100%, then you are:

2. Aspiring toward the raw food diet

3. You eat more raw food than cooked.

2 & 3 are both healthier than the Standard American Diet,

but 100% is "the Ideal."

S.A.D. Diet: Standard American Degenerative Diet. Predominantly cooked & processed food which includes meat, dairy, flour, sugar, refined oils, condiments, spices & junk food. Very, very sad, indeed!**Sproutarian:** Sproutarians eat mainly sprouts or only sprouts including sprouted grains, legumes, nuts & seeds. Young sprouts are an extremely rejuvenative food, so sproutarians tend to be very strong and vital.

Sunfoods: This term expresses the idea that the ideal foods are found undisturbed, in the state of nature, and are brimming with positive energy from the sun which they impart to us when we eat them.

Toxemia: Saturation of the body with toxins which come from both exogenous and endogenous sources. Toxemia is the one cause of all disease.

Vital Force: Solar energy we absorb from the raw food we eat, the water we drink, and the air we breathe. Vital force is also replenished by securing adequate rest and sleep. Also called Life Force, Vital Magnetism, Nerve Energy, Prana, Orgone Energy, Odic Force, Vrill.

Vitarian: A Fruitarian who will not eat nuts or seeds. Vitarians believe nuts & seeds were the "forbidden fruit" in the Garden of Eden which caused us to fall from a state of godlike immortality to our present condition. They believe a strict diet of low protein, water-rich fruits & vegetables with austere spiritual devotion can restore us to our original purity. They use a unique type of fasting: the Aquarian Tinctured Water Regimen - in which 1% fruit juice is added to 99% water to dissolve mucoid plaque from the intestines which they claim regular fasting cannot do. The main proponent of Vitarianism was the late Dr. Johnny Lovewisdo, who lived in the mountains of Ecuador and claimed to be the reincarnation of John the Baptist. He was once found living in the crater of an extinct volcano in the Andes, having gone without food for a period of over 7 months, in a state of ecstasy. He practiced his regimen for many decades beginning in the 1940's. He was a true fearless trailblazer, yet in the later years of his life, he suffered from poor health as a result of the lingering effects of a previous exposure to pesticide poisoning, over-eating raw foods and bingeing on cooked foods. Lovewisdom contributed many valuable ideas to the evolution of raw food eating, but he has paid heavily in later years for his fearless experimentation. Extreme caution is advised for those who wish to try this most extreme form of raw food vegetarianism. Anthropologists at John's Hopkins University showed that ancient humans did at one time subsist solely on fruits but that may be because the fruit in those days was still mineral-rich as a result of glacial mineral dust spread over the planet by receding glaciers of the out-going of the last Ice Age.

Water: Water should be free from the poisonous inorganic minerals. Use only distilled water for this reason. Water-rich fruit contains only the life-giving organic minerals; therefore fruit is said to be nature's perfect distiller. The water in fruits is structured water, filled with the purifying energy of the Sun. Some fruitarians who live in unpolluted areas drink rain water. Coconut water is also very good.

Wild Foods: Many of the fruits & vegetables we eat today have been hybridized by man and bear little resemblance to the original   versions of these same foods on which our ancestors thrived for millions of years. Many of these foods are too high in sugars and have other nutritional imbalances. When we eat wild raw foods as they are found in nature, we eat foods that our bodies are genetically encoded for. Our bodies can use them efficiently, with a minimum of waste. They reconnect us with the wild natural spiritual energy of the land which gave us our bodies in the first place. Anyone can learn to identify & forage for wild foods which are available for free!

Thanks to Habib Baily for this dictionary.

RAW READING

Recommended Reading & References

Against The Grain by Jax Peters Lowell

Amazing New Health System—The Inner Clean Way by Morris Krok

Be Your Own Doctor by Ann Wigmore

Become Younger by Norman Walker

Better Eyesight Without Glasses by William Bates

Better Sight Without Glasses by Harry Benjamin

Beyond Beef by Jeremy Rafkin

Blatant Raw Foodist Propaganda by Joe Alexander

Bragg Healthy Lifestyle, Vital Living to 120!
by Paul and Patricia Bragg

Conscious Eating by Dr. Gabriel Cousens

Children of the Sun by Gordon Kennedy

Dining In the Raw by Rita Romano (Raw recipe book)

Eco-Eating by Sopoty Brook

Enzyme Nutrition by Dr. Edward Howell

Fasting Can Save Your Life by Herbert Shelton

Fasting For Health And Long Life
by Hereward Carrington

Feel Good Food by Karen Knowler & Susie Miller

Fit For Life by Harvey & Marilyn Diamond

Food Combining Made Easy by Dr. Herbert Shelton

Food For The Gods by Rynn Berry

Fruit Can Heal You by Dr. O.L.M. Abramowski

Fruit The Food And Medicine For Man by Morris Krok

Grain Damage by Douglas Graham

Hooked On Raw by Rhio

How To Improve Your Eyes by Margaret Darst Corbett

Identifying and Harvesting Edible and Medicinal Plants
by Steve Brill

Instinctive Nutrition by Severen L Schaeffer

Is Menstruation Necessary?
by Wendy Harris and Nadine Forrest Mac Donald

Ishmael by Daniel Quinn

Living Foods For Optimum Health by Brian Clement

Many Lives, Many Masters by Brian Weiss

Man's Higher Consciousness by Hilton Hotema

Mucusless Diet Healing System by Arnold Ehret

Mutant Message Down Under by Margo Morgan

Nature's First Law: The Raw Food Diet
by Arlin, Dini and Wolfe

Nutrition and Athletic Performance by Douglas Graham

Peace Pilgrim by Friends of the Peace Pilgrim

Perfect Body by Roe Gallo

Primal Mothering In A Modern World by Hygeia Halfmoon

Rational Fasting by Arnold Ehret

Raw Power by Steve Arlin

Relearn To See by Thomas R. Quackenbush

Rhino Resources by Scott Alexander

Survival Into The 21st Century by Viktoras Kulvinskas

Sweet Temptations by Frances Kendall (Raw recipe book)

Toxemia Explained by John Tilden

The Children's Health Food Book by Ron Seaborn

The Fruits Of Healing by Dave Klein

The Great Exotic Fruit Book by Norman Van Aken

The Hippocrates Diet by Ann Wigmore

The Language Crystal by Lawrence William Lyons

The Miracle Of Fasting by Paul Bragg

The Raw Truth by Jeremy Safron & Renee Underkoffler (Raw recipe book)

The Sunfood Diet Success System by Dave Wolfe

The Sunfood Way to Health Dugald Semple

The Treasury Of Quotes by Jim Rohn

Vegan Nutrition: Pure and Simple by Michael Klaper

Vibrant Living by Natalie Cederquist & James Levin (Raw recipe book)

Your Natural Diet: Alive Raw Foods
by David Klein and T.C. Fry

Why Suffer? by Ann Wigmore

RAW ORGANIZATIONS AND RESOURCES

Raw Life
Paul Nison
P.O. Box 996
New York, NY 10002
917-506-1124 (pager)
Web Site: http://www.rawlife.com
E-mail: paul@rawlife.com

Nature's First Law
P.O. Box 900202
San Diego, CA 92190 USA
619-645-7282
800-205-2350-orders
Web Site: http://www.rawfood.com
E-mail: nature@io-online.com

Nature's First Law is The World's Premier Source of Raw-Food Diet Books, Juicers, Videos, and Audio tapes.

Living Nutrition Magazine
P.O. Box 256
Sebastopol, California 95473-256
707-887-9132
Web Site: http://www.livingnutrition.com
E-mail: dave@livingnutrition.com
The World's premier magazine dedicated to helping
health seekers learn how to succeed with
eating our natural diet of raw foods!

Doug Graham
305-743-8882
Dr. Graham is a world-renowned health and performance
coach. Call Doug to inquire about his services or for
lecture information, coaching, videos, books, charts
plus much more information.

Dr. Tim Trader
305-703-4405
If you need a natural doctor's advice, I would recommend
you call Dr. Tim Trader. He lives in Hawaii but will take calls
from anywhere in the United States.

Dr. Fred Bisci
718-979-7950
The best nutritionist in the world!
His office in located in Staten Island New York

Roe Gallo
P.O. Box 25512
San Mateo CA 94402
Web Site: http://www.roegallo.com
Author of: Body Ecology, Perfect Body, Beyond the Matrix

Gil Jacobs
Chakra 17
New York City
212-679-6576
Web Site: http://www.Chakra17.com
For questions or information about
colonic therapy contact Gil.

Planet Health
Ed Leib
18 East 23rd Street
New York, NY 10010
212-253-2262
800-398-6237
Web Site: http://www.ehealth.htmlplanet.com/
E-mail: planethealth@mail.com
Produces a television program about
living naturally called "Accent On Wellness."
Also a major distributor of rebounders.

Glaser Farms
Stan Glaser
191000 SW 137 Ave.
Miami, FL 33177
305-238-7747
Fax 305-238-1227
Organic Growers* Distributors * Dehydrators
Organic Produce, Tropical Fruit, Dried Fruit
and Natural Food Products

Rhio's Raw Energy Hotline
212-343-1152
Raw and living foods information in
New York City and worldwide

Wild Food Information
Steve Brill
718-291-6825
E-mail: wildmansteve@bigfoot.com
Steve is the most knowledgeable naturalist
in the U.S. He leads wild food and
ecology tours throughout the Northeast.

Essence of Health Books
Susan Krok
211 Bean Creek
Scotts Valley, Calfornia 95006
Web Site: http://www.essenceofhealth.net
E-mail: susan@susiekdigital.com
To order a catalogue of all of Morris Krok's
books and other great hard-to-find writings
on the raw food diet, contact Susan.

fresh network
P.O. Box 71
ELY, CAMBS, CB7 4GU, UK
+44-0-8708-00-7070
Web Site: http://www.fresh-network.com
E-mail: info@fresh-network.com
Raw food information in the UK and an excellent
raw food magazine

Aris La Tham
House Of Life,
Jamaica
To contact Aris call Rainbow Travel
Linda Horton
877-67-RELAX
Live food classes and retreat

Loving Foods
Jeremy Safron
P.O. Box 576
Paia HI, 96779
310-RAW-FOOD
Web Site: http://www.lovingfoods.com
E-mail: allraw@lovingfoods.com
Raw Merchandise, Information, Publishing, Consulting

Ann Wigmore Institute
P.O. Box 429
Rincon, P.R. 00677
787-868-6307

Hippocrates Health Institute
1443 Palmdale Court
West Palm Beach, FL 33411
800-842-2125
561-471-8876

Optimum Health Institute
6970 Central Ave.
Lemon Grove, CA 91945
619-646-3346

Batista Mini Market
Luis Batista
120 Essex Street
New York NY, 10002
A great N.Y.C. Spanish produce market for baby coconuts.

Caravan of Dreams
405 East 6th Street
New York, NY 10009
212-254-1613
Caravan offers vegan cuisine and raw-food dishes. They
also host seminars and lectures.

Quintessence
263 East 10th Street
New York NY, 10009
646-654-1823
The only 100% Raw-Food restaurant in NYC
100% Organic and 100% Raw

Fertility Awareness Center
Barbara Feldman
P.O. Box 2606
New York, NY 10009
212-475-4490
E-mail: bleaf@usa.net
Learn birth control—the natural way. Barbara will teach
you the natural way to prevent pregnancy with out taking
any drugs. This is not the Rhythm Method. It is done by
knowing which days in each cycle you are not fertile.
Call Barbara to find out more.

Illustrations
Tom Cushwa
212-228-2615
E-mail: Cushwa@panix.com

Forward Studio
Art Direction & Graphic Design
Enrique Candioti
E-mail: forward@interport.net

Eco Books
192 Fifth Avenue
Brooklyn, NY 11217
718-623-2698
E-mail: treichler@ecobooks.com
New York's Environmental Bookstore

Vita-Mix Blenders
Evergreen Trade
Terry Dreisewerd
17321 Irvine Blvd. #100
Tustin, CA 92780
800-422-7980
Web Site: http://www.evergreentrade.com
The best prices for a Vita-Mix blender! Mention this book
"The Raw Life" and receive a special discount

Hygeia Center
18 East 23rd Street
New York, NY 10010
800-525-7973
Health, Empowerment, Educational, Community Center

Living and raw foods comunity
John Kohler
Web Site http://www.living-foods.com
The world's largest community bulletin board on the
internet educating people on the value of raw foods.

Raw Food Appliances
John Kohler
Web Site: http://www.discountjuicers.com
Offering raw food appliances, dehydrators, juicers,
sprouters and water distillers, shower filters at discount
prices, including informative articles to learn more about
juicers, along with video demonstrations of the juicers.

Raw Foods Network in Portland
Habib Baily
1538 SE 122 Ave #49
Protland, Oregon 97233
503-256-8351
Web Site: http://www.users.uswest.net/~rawimmortal/index.html
E-mail: rawimmortal@home.net
Raw Food events, classes, food prep and more.
If your in Portland contact Habib

Health Research
P.O. Box 850
Pomeroy, WA 99347
888-844-2386
Web Site: http://www.healthresearchbooks.com
Publishers of rare and out-of-print books
Nutritional Reasearch, Natural Healing, Health,
Metaphysics, religion, esoterica.
Over 2,000 listings in more than 130 Categories!
Many of the quotes from the chapters of this book
were taken from books offered by Health Research. Con-
tact them to order these and other great books.

High Vibe Health and Healing
85 East 3rd Street
New York, NY 10003
888-554-6645
Web Site: http://www.highvibe.com
They sell live food vitamins and minerals, herbs and herbal formulas, pure organic oils, books, air and water purifiers, juicers and live food staples

The Raw Truth Cafe and Wellness Center
Bob Saladino
3620 East Flamingo Road
Las Vegas, Nevada, 89121
702-450-9007
Web Site: http://www.rawfoodist.com/rawtruth
E-mail: therawtruthlv@hotmail.com
100% Organic and 100% Raw food restaurant in Las Vegas

Dentist
Dr. Bill Busch
2000 Swift Avenue
North Kansas City, MO 64116
816-471-2911
Web Site: http://www.drbusch.com
E-mail: drbusch@kc.rr.com
Worth the trip to Kansas City to get your mercury fillings removed or any other dental work you need.

The Date People
P.O. Box 808
Niland, CA 92257
E-mail: datefolk@brawleyonline.com
Growing certified organic soft dates

Colitis & Crohn's Health Recovery Services
Dave Klein
707-887-9132
Web Site: http://www.colitis-crohns.com
E-mail: dave@colitis-crohns.com
Teaching the natural way to self heal IBD and create
everlasting wellness

Healthful Living International
Web Site: http://www.healthgeniuses.com
The world's premiere Natural Hygiene organization

Arnold's Way
Raw Cafe
4438 Main Street
Philadelphia, PA 19127
215-483-2266
100% Raw food Cafe that specializes in bananas
They sell Banana Whips-Soup-Pies-Cakes-Bars
-Smoothies & Shakes

ORDER FORM

THE RAW LIFE: BECOMING NATURAL IN AN UNNATURAL WORLD
PLEASE SEND ME ___ COPIES AT **US$ 19.95 PER COPY**

THE RAW LIFE AUDIO CASSETTE
PLEASE SEND ME ___ AUDIO TAPES AT *US$ 9.95 PER TAPE*

THE RAW LIFE VIDEO
PLEASE SEND ME _____ VIDEO TAPES AT US$ **14.95 PER VIDEO**

US Shipping and Handling:
$3.50 per first item, $1.00 for each additional item
International Shipping and Handling:
$6.00 per first item, $2.00 for each additional item

TOTAL AMOUNT ENCLOSED $_____

SHIP TO:
Please print

NAME _____

ADDRESS_____

City_____STATE_____

ZIP CODE_____COUNTRY_____

EMAIL ADDRESS_____

PHONE NUMBER_____

Please copy or cut out this form and mail with a check, money order or bank draft in US currency payable to:

Paul Nison
P.O. Box 996
New York, NY 10002

To contact the author e-mail:paul@rawlife.com
Or go to: website: http://www.rawlife.com

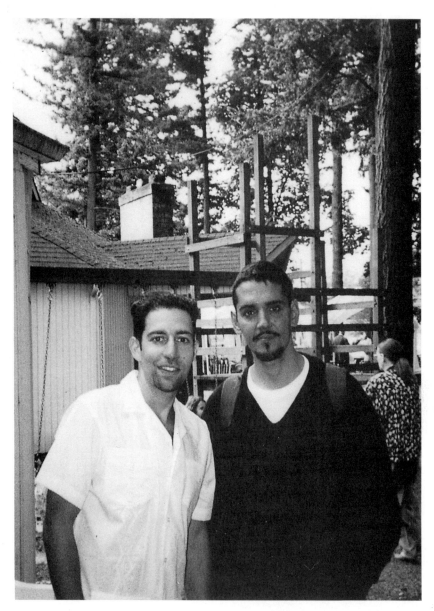

Paul Nison a.k.a. "The Durian King" and Enrique Candioti a.k.a. "Raw Hermit" living the raw life—and thriving!